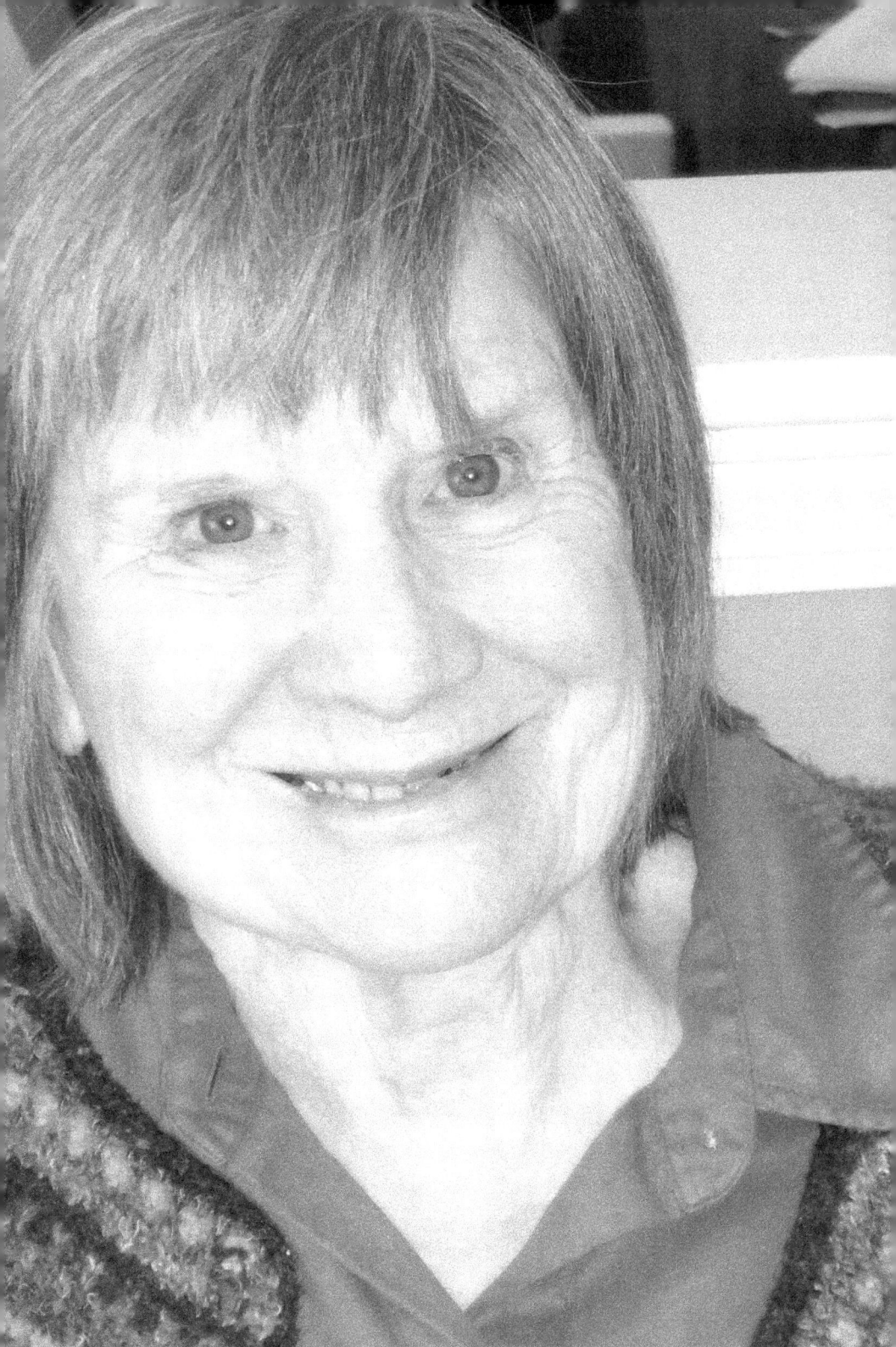

Molly now.

What Do I Do Now?
A Caregiver's Journey with Alzheimer's

Willem O'Reilly

Kenosis Publishing

Lafayette, Colorado

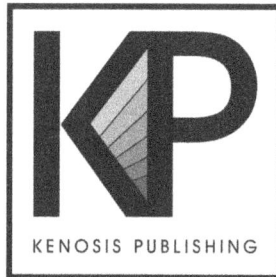

KENOSIS PUBLISHING

For permission requests, write to the publisher at the address below.

Kenosis Publishing
455 Strathmore Lane #212
Lafayette, CO 80026
www.willemor917writer.com

Printed in the United States of America

ISBN 9780996543507

LOC Control Number
2015913152

First Edition
14 13 12 11 10 9 8 7 6 5 4 3 2 1

Edited by Mary Ellen Byrne

Designed by Reynor O'Reilly

Photos by Willem O'Reilly

This book is dedicated to Molly.

To Bernadette, Zoe, and Beth and Karl.

Life changing experiences can move us to pass along what we believe we have learned. We want to shout about a birth to the heavens. We want to place the face of someone we have lost in the stars. We want people to know.

Scott Simon

Unforgettable: A Son, A Mother, and the Lessons of a Lifetime

What Do I Do Now?
A Caregiver's Journey with Alzheimer's

Table of Contents

Part Two: New Normal

Part Three: The Long Road

Part Four: Meditations

Introduction

Molly, my wife of over thirty years, has Alzheimer's. Presently, Alzheimer's is terminal, untreatable, and incurable. Barring a catastrophic injury, such as a fall that breaks her hip, Molly will die of Alzheimer's—she will die from the continual shutting down of her brain cells until her body ceases to function. This, then, is fundamentally a book about Molly's declining towards death and about my coping with the grief of losing her bit-by-bit.

Who is the Molly I was grieving?

There is a scene in the stage adaptation of the book *Still Alice* in which Alice, who has early onset Alzheimer's, is looking at a book that she co-wrote years earlier with her husband. She says, "This seems familiar." He replies, "It should. We wrote it together. . . . You are the smartest person I ever knew."

I say this often about Molly. She is indeed the smartest person I have ever known: Phi Beta Kappa at Stanford and Ph.D. from Princeton. She was, in fact, only the third woman to receive a Ph.D. in English from Princeton University. During her long career as a Professor of English, Molly published in top journals and lectured at conferences in the U.S., Canada, and Europe.

For many years Molly taught English composition using the text of *Zen and the Art of Motorcycle Maintenance* by Robert Pirsig. When a volume was published on how to teach the book, her approach was featured as particularly exemplary.

These are some of the bare bones items from her curriculum vitae. There was much, much more. She was, for example, also fluent in Italian. When we went to dinner in Rome the waiter flirted with her after she ordered in a perfect accent and I spoke my adult education travel Italian. "What are you doing with this idiot?" the waiter asked. "You deserve better."

Very true: Molly deserved only the best. There were very few people who could match her intelligence, education, integrity, loyalty, perseverance, work ethic, and generosity.

Preface

This is both a book about Alzheimer's and not about Alzheimer's. At the beginning of writing it, I thought it was all about this terrible disease and its effects on the woman I love.

Around 2006 Molly started losing her abilities, and I began taking over for her. Molly's last job was tutoring master's degree nursing students online. As she declined, she had trouble with the computing. Many tasks, such as logging on, downloading, and saving documents with a new name, became too much for her. I helped with those.

She could, however, still tell where a comma belonged, whether a subject agreed with the verb, what words or phrases required hyphens. After over thirty-five years, the principles of grammar and composition were deeply ingrained in her memory.

I was amazed at how long they lasted.

Molly had become aware of her diminished capabilities, and she went to see her doctor. Even without a definite diagnosis, the local doctor suspected the onset of dementia and prescribed Aricept, the standard medication that is supposed to slow down the progress of Alzheimer's disease. At first, Molly kept her concerns and her medication a secret, even from me. However, it soon became evident to both of us that something was seriously wrong.

In late 2007, we went together to see another physician, Dr. Amatelli, who put Molly through the standard protocol: test for thyroid function; then test for evidence of small strokes. After eliminating these possibilities, he ordered an MRI, which can reveal the spaces created by the nerve tangles in the brain that specifically indicate Alzheimer's. The MRI showed evidence of just such holes.

After Dr. Amatelli's careful procedure, we were pretty confident of the diagnosis, but we consulted an expert at the university medical center to be certain. Yes, indeed, the MRI showed conclusive evidence of Alzheimer's. This consultation, in February of 2008, confirmed that Molly had Alzheimer's.

That is only part of the story. This book has turned out to be just as much about my journey as a caregiver. For five years I was wholly enmeshed in caring for Molly at home: that was my primary purpose, trumping all other aspects of life. I had no time or energy for, or interest in, much of anything else. If I ever had a choice of doing something for or with Molly or other-wise, I always chose Molly first.

When I had to let go of caring for Molly full time and turn her over to professional caregivers in 2012, I was devastated. If there were a YouTube video of me that morning, it would show me in front of the memory-care facility sobbing uncontrollably. I felt nothing but overt grief: loss, sadness, and failure.

For the past two years, while I was writing what follows, I have been experiencing what has been labeled "anticipatory grief." Since Molly is still alive, my grieving for her now is not exactly the same as grieving for a person who has died. Still, my anticipatory grief is real: it still hurts and is some-times overwhelming.

Grieving is a process that takes time. Many people, especially in our can-do culture, believe that it is best to grieve for a relatively short period and then to get on with life. However, those who work directly with the bereaved now say that a two-year grieving period is normal and healthy.

These essays, then, are my journal of grieving the Molly I have known for over thirty years. My smart, funny, strong, generous, kind, sweet Molly is no longer fully present. I grieved every time I wanted to share something with her and realized that she could not understand what I was telling her. She had no memory at all of who she was and what we did together. She didn't remember my name or the names of her children.

Writing down my thoughts and feelings became my personal coping strategy. It was only after I began creating these essays that friends and family started saying to me, "There are so many people who are going through the same things you are. Alzheimer's is everywhere now. What you are writing can be helpful to others."

Because I wrote for myself, often in an emotional state, my pieces are raw in terms of style. However, my coaches and supporters, many of whom know much more about the craft of writing than I do, say that my directness is an advantage. I may be able to communicate what other caregivers think and feel and are yet unable to articulate, or perhaps reluctant to express.

Willem O'Reilly
Lafayette, Colorado

Part One: Coping

MEN WHO CARE

December 23, 2012

I am a caregiver. And I am a man.

My wife Molly, who has Alzheimer's, is in a facility now. I still visit her every day. Before she was admitted three months ago, I was a full-time caregiver for five years.

Over these years I have come to realize that caregiving requires some manly virtues: strength, courage, loyalty. Of course, it also requires some traditionally feminine virtues: sensitivity, compassion, self-sacrifice.

I've learned to employ all of these virtues and more.

I have, for example, learned much about courage. Courage is not about not being afraid. Rather it is about feeling the fear and acting anyway. When Molly was behaving in a psychotic way, it meant being with her instead of running away. I learned that I had a much greater capacity for courage than I ever thought possible.

Indeed, Molly's Alzheimer's has challenged me to use all of my experience, all of my skills, all of my tools, many of which I never knew I had. Others I had to develop as we went along.

I am more patient now; I've had to learn to be. There is no point in getting frustrated when things take "too long," or when Molly can't understand what I am asking her to do.

My communication skills are much more advanced now. I truly understand how important body language is, how important touch is, how important active listening is.

I also have come to recognize the importance of emotion in communication. When I am calm and peaceful, the channels are open not blocked. When I am agitated, Molly and I have trouble connecting.

Although not always obvious, new modes of communication can be learned. Over time I have observed and learned what works and what doesn't.

Molly is different now: there are things (like reading and writing) that she can't do anymore. There are other signs of the late stages of the disease, like incontinence. But I still know her at the most fundamental level. She is still Molly. She is still the woman I married twenty-eight years ago.

I now carry her memories, remember her stories. It makes me feel very sad and very privileged at the same time. I know her. I remember what she cannot. I appreciate the life we have led, the things we did together. I recall them when I am with her. I share them with her when she cannot remember herself. This sharing brings us moments of happiness and joy. These are precious.

Have I given up myself to care for Molly? No, not really. It is true that living with Alzheimer's has made my life different. I have changed; I have developed; I have grown.

And I am more virtuous: I am more manly not less. I am stronger, more courageous, more loyal than ever before. I have been challenged to the depth of my being, and I have risen to the challenge. I was overwhelmed, but I more than survived. I am a better man.

TERMINAL, UNTREATABLE, INCURABLE

My wife Molly has Alzheimer's, a terminal, untreatable, incurable disease.

Untreatable? That's not right: We treat all kinds of serious conditions now. I had prostate cancer. I had an operation. Ever since, my PSA has been "undetectable." The treatment worked.

With Alzheimer's the doctors said, "Medications may slow it down, but there is no cure."

For years I lived in denial. Molly would be different. I thought, "Molly is very smart: She was Phi Beta Kappa at Stanford and earned a Ph.D. in English at Princeton. Her brain is more powerful, more adaptable, more resilient.

All that didn't matter. Five years after her diagnosis, she exhibited the same symptoms of decline as other Alzheimer's patients. She couldn't read or write. She couldn't remember her phone number. She wandered. She spit out her food like a small child. She was incontinent. When she took the thirty-point cognitive functioning test at the neurologist, she scored a frightening three.

I got in the habit of responding to the question, "And what do you do?" with "I am a full-time caregiver." It was true because Molly needed assistance with almost all of the "activities of daily living."

Later I arranged for limited respite periods. I got my fourteen hours a week respite to "take care of myself." I laugh now at the thought that such a scheme could possibly be sufficient for anyone dealing with 24/7 caregiving.

What was I trying to prove? You and I both know the answer: "I am strong; I am a competent adult; I am a problem solver; I am good in a crisis; I can handle this by myself." What nonsense we tell ourselves!

Luckily I did have several voices of sanity in my life as well. First there was my sister Bernadette, a trained therapist, who teaches adult education for the Los Angeles County Schools. Bern just happened to be teaching a course for caregivers of the elderly with dementia. I would call her two or three times a week and say, "This just happened." Or, "Molly just did this." "What do I do now?" and Bern would reply, "Well, you could try . . ." Or, "I'm not sure, but I'll find out for you."

Bern's go-to source for additional information about Alzheimer's and caregiving was Stefanie Elkins, then Director of Leeza's Place, a center for caregiver support. Between Bern and Stefanie I had excellent information and advice about the whole range of problems and challenges I was facing.

I also had support from my sponsor and friends in my Al-Anon Twelve Step group. Many of them stepped forward during my recovery from surgery and helped out in many ways with Molly. Indeed, when it was no longer safe for Molly to be left home alone for any period of time, I took her with me to my meetings on Friday evenings and the group dinners afterward. All the members of the group got to know Molly. They knew of her illness and were very kind when she commented or wandered or ate with her fingers.

I had help from the caregivers sent by the agency and, later, from my friend Beth. Beth had worked in caregiving for the elderly previously, and she offered to sign on again with her old agency and take on Molly's respite care schedule. Beth watched Molly for fourteen hours each week, and I put in the other 154.

Often Beth was the only person other than Molly I would see on any given day, and we became very close friends. In fact Beth was the one who went with me when I took Molly to the facility.

That was the critical existential moment for me. When Molly exhibited behavior that mimicked psychosis, I realized I could no longer care for her at home and meet her needs. It was crushing to lose my life's purpose. If I couldn't take care of the person I loved most in the world, then what was I good for?

IT'S TIME

When I could no longer maintain my denial, I came face-to-face with decisions I didn't want to make. The most upsetting was the "when": When would she get so bad that I couldn't take care of her at home anymore?

I began the placement process: I went to a local conference on elder care. I collected brochures from respite care agencies. I consulted with her and our children, with my psychiatrist, and with my therapist sister. I even visited some memory-care units and talked to them about daycare. I was ready, so I thought.

Meanwhile, Molly had become more aggressive. She hit and kicked her respite caregiver. Her incontinence was getting worse.

I was getting worse, too—worn down and out by the constant vigilance and the constant rushes of adrenalin when she did something unsafe, like trimming her fingernails with a steak knife. I was exhausted.

She began to have episodes in which she was completely out of touch with reality. Then one evening, she stripped naked, stood at the window in our spare bedroom, and yelled "Stop!" at the tennis players on the court below. I could do nothing to reach her, nothing to comfort her.

It was time.

Time for me to take Molly to a facility.   Not next year but now.

I contacted her insurance company and found out about her benefits. When they confirmed her coverage, I called the facility and made an appointment to sign the paperwork.

This was the hardest decision I have ever made. And, despite all the advice and support I got, I had to make it alone. And live with it.

It was necessary for Molly's safety and well-being, and for my own. So I acted in our best interests. Still, I felt guilty. It will take a long, long time to get over that feeling.

FIRST DAY

On Molly's first day, we arrived at the appointed time at the memory-care facility, but there was no one there to meet us. Not a good start. Molly's son Chris and her respite caregiver Beth had come to help out. The plan had been to get a staff member to distract Molly at the front of the building while we brought her things in through the back door.

Beth and I had taken her there for music events so she'd know the place ahead of time, but we had never left her there alone. Once inside, Molly sensed that something was going on and started to get agitated. No staff person was available to even try to distract her.

As soon as Chris and I went out to the car to bring things in, Molly started racing around the building looking for us. It's a rather small place—room for fifty-two residents—so she found us in her new room in no time. She burst in with a staff nurse trailing helplessly behind. We had to leave the room with her and defer the unpacking until later.

All three of us took turns walking Molly around the facility for the next half hour. Eventually, Chris got her to calm down and sit with him in the lounge. Meanwhile, I unpacked her clothing and personal items and went outside to cry.

The sobs overtook me, and my body convulsed. For a few moments, my senses partially shut down. I saw nothing and heard only my own gasps.

This is what is meant, I suppose, when we say that we feel with our hearts. Intense feelings are not things of the mind: they are not thoughts. They come from a place where thinking "I am sad" or "I am lonely" is completely inadequate.

In a few minutes Beth joined me, and we drove away. I knew beforehand that I would be in no condition to drive so she took the wheel. When we got to her house, I collapsed. It was only 11:00 in the morning, but I was exhausted.

About five hours later I received a call from the Director. She shocked me by saying, "This has been the worst day I've had in my ten years here." Apparently, Molly had been highly upset all day, running around the unit and going into all the rooms that weren't locked.

"She's too quick for us. And we're concerned that she may knock down some of the older residents. It's a safety issue." "I understand," I responded automatically. "Some of the care partners are afraid of her," the Director continued. "But how can that be?" I said. "She only weighs 125 pounds." "Some of our care partners are even smaller."

In my head I'm thinking, "Oh, no, they're going to kick her out the first day. I've planned for this for weeks and gotten my courage up to do it today. I have no plan B. What am I going to do?"

TWO PERCENT LEFT AND SUICIDAL THOUGHTS

Right before Molly went into the memory-care facility, my sister Bernadette commented that I had "about 2% left." I don't know how she came up with the number, but Bernadette was right on about my being very near total exhaustion.

I didn't think my situation could be as dire as all that. After all, I had respite care four afternoons a week. Molly still went to bed at a reasonable hour and slept through the night. So, I was getting a "good night's sleep."

What I had no awareness of then was how exhausting the waking hours had become. I was always on alert trying to keep Molly safe and constantly anxious about what might happen next. For example, we battled about her getting out of the car when the respite person came, and she made a scene whenever I left the house. I rode the emotional waves with her, sometimes up in the air and sometimes crashing on the shore.

Among Molly's newest symptoms was hyperactivity. One manifestation was her insisting that we go somewhere in the car. As we started out, Molly would point the way as though she had a destination in mind, but soon she would become confused and lost. Apparently, she just felt compelled to be out of the house and moving. Where we went mattered little.

All of this was taking a toll I could not comprehend.

In the process of deciding when Molly needed to go to the facility, I had lots of good advice and support. Everyone told me I needed to "take care of myself." Fortunately for me, I had learned to ask for help during my treatment for cancer two years previously (the surgery was successful and I am cancer free).

Thus, when I took Molly to the facility, I arranged to stay with my 12 Step sponsor and his wife for a week. I was safe there. While I was with them, I felt surprisingly calm, though I was very sad.

The first week without Molly ended on my birthday. I spent the evening with Molly's son Chris, his wife Bethany, and Molly's grandchildren Brian and Matthew. I figured I'd be OK to go home after the cake and singing "Happy Birthday." I was.

Next morning, however, I found myself in the kitchen starting to prepare breakfast. I realized I didn't even know the measurements for one serving of oatmeal instead of two, and I broke down.

About thirty-six hours later, I hit my lowest point.

I thought, "This is too painful. I am too tired to do this anymore. If I were gone, Molly's sons, Chris and Reynor, could take care of whatever she still needed. My job is done. I could just take an overdose of pills and go to sleep."

This must have been when a Higher Power intervened because I am still here writing this.

MAD AT GOD

Alzheimer's, like alcoholism, is a disease that affects both the patient and the caregiver in every way: physically, emotionally, psychologically, and spiritually.

As to the latter, my reaction to the disease has been pretty straightforward. I was mad at God, the Creator, Master of the Universe. I thought it was terribly unjust that a beautiful, loving, intelligent woman should be so afflicted. What is the lesson to be learned from such suffering? What a waste.

But this dilemma raises a problem. If I'm mad at God, then God knows I'm mad at Him, and I'm going to get punished for the sin of anger. That engenders fear and anxiety, which can block out all other feelings—even positive ones. So it's an uncomfortable place to be.

However, that's exactly where I found myself in the weeks after I took Molly to the memory-care facility. Whenever anyone mentioned Molly's spirit or God's plan, I couldn't take comfort in it. I was just pissed off. Later I came to some acceptance of Molly's condition. Part of the evolution of my thinking and feeling comes from my experience over many years with Twelve Step programs. Steps Two and Three, in particular, are God steps. Step Two states "Came to believe that a power greater than ourselves [usually referred to as a Higher Power] could restore us to sanity."

Three reads, "Made a decision to turn our will and our lives over to the care of God as we understood God." The Twelve Step programs are based on the belief that there is a Higher Power who helps us.

I can say that I'm now willing to believe that God, as I understand God, is not out to get me or punish me through Molly. Still I have trouble with "turning our lives over to the *care* of God."

Does God, the Creator of the Universe, really care about Molly and me? Most of the time, that does not seem at all likely.

The twelve steps are intentionally written in the past tense. They articulate the actual experiences of real people who have gone through the process they describe. Some people who have been where I am now have come to believe in a caring God. That means I can, too. It may take time, maybe a long time, but there is Hope.

LONELINESS

After only four months, fourteen days, and about one hour, I finally realized I could not escape the loneliness. I counted the time from when I took Molly to the memory-care unit on September 10, 2012 at 9:30 a.m.

In the ensuing days, there were plenty of distractions. My family of origin was good for at least a crisis a month, maybe one a week. The drama is often entertaining, even exhilarating. It's life and death around there: my Mother is eighty-eight and fragile, and she's already had one very close call. There's madness and sanity: I have several schizophrenic relatives, especially an adopted son, whose behavior and situation are endlessly unpredictable. There's also prosperity and ruin: Six of my siblings have jobs with benefits, a pretty good measure of security. But seven of my siblings and myself do not.

Still, distractions are not enough to escape the loneliness.

Well, what about friends? Activities? Groups? They're supposed to help, and they do sometimes. I go out to lunch, attend movies and musical performances, host small dinner parties. I attend a Buddhist meditation group and belong to a book club at the public library. I go to a 12 Step meeting every Friday evening. I participate in A Course in Miracles. In fact, I'm usually booked five nights a week.

Yet, keeping busy doesn't allow me to escape the loneliness.

Grandchildren. Now that must surely do the trick. I have two for sure and possibly a third (but that's a long story). There's also another one on the way. When I'm with the one who's three and a half, I'm engaged and happy. But he tests limits and drives his parents crazy, and I have to bite my tongue and not interfere.

So, even a new generation won't let me escape the loneliness for long.

Art and creativity? I still take pictures. I love images of nature, and living in Colorado provides me with endless photogenic beauty in the sky, mountains, forests, and flowered meadows. Molly and I used to hike all summer, and I'd always take my camera. I have "captured" many stunning scenes.

I've taken fewer art photographs lately. Now, I'm more focused on people and a record. Memories seem so ephemeral. I want something concrete I can hold in my hand. "Here's a picture of Molly and me in the Tuilleries Gardens in Paris. See. It really happened."

Thus, art doesn't let me escape the loneliness.

It might help to know what goes on in Molly's mind. Does she know she's married? Does she know she has two sets of kids and double-digit grandchildren? Does she know she is a native Angelino? Does she know that Italian was her second language? Does she know she was a professor and taught everything from Milton to *Zen and the Art of Motorcycle Maintenance?* I'd like to know what she knows, but I don't and I can't.

And so, whatever is left inside won't help me escape the loneliness.

It's a cliché–but probably one of those that's based in truth—that every one of us dies alone. And only then do we escape the loneliness.

GUILT AND SHAME

My friend Beth says that I can feel guilty about anything. It's an automatic reaction to a wide variety of events. Well, I've worked hard at feeling guilty, and I've gotten quite good at it over a lifetime.

When I was a child in parochial school, we had a complete curriculum in guilt. We were taught to feel guilty about Godless communism in Russia—I guess we weren't praying hard enough. We also learned guilt about the starving children in India and China—not to mention the poor pagan babies in Africa who had no access to church or sacraments. And, of course, the really big guilt was for the sufferings of Jesus, caused—so we were told—largely by our lying to our sainted mothers and our other heinous crimes.

Therapists and self-help authors say it's very important to make the distinction between guilt and shame. There's a common formula that goes, "Guilt means you *made* a mistake. Shame means you *are* a mistake."

Making a mistake presumes you can correct it and move on beyond it. Shame you always carry with you.

So, I've been confused about how I feel regarding putting Molly in the unit. Sometimes it seems like a guilty mistake: I got the timing wrong or the place wrong. Or, I underestimated Molly's capacities for activities of daily living. Mistakes any reasonable person might make under the circumstances.

Other times, it feels like shame. If I were a better person, if I were more determined, if I loved Molly more, if I weren't so selfish, I could have kept her at home.

Lately, I've been thinking a lot about finances. And the bottom line is that Molly's insurance and pension will both run out in about three years. Then what? She's healthy physically, no heart problems or diabetes. She may live a long time. So, when the money is gone, does she go to a place with few resources where the patients sit around in wheelchairs drooling?

That doesn't sound right (and, yes, I do know that this is all irrational speculation about the unknown future). But I've fantasized about bringing her home again, because, of course, I "would have no choice." Thus, I could redeem myself for my failures.

That looks like shame to me. It says there is something fundamentally wrong with me. I didn't just make an understandable mistake: I was inadequate, not up to the challenges of life.

I've been through enough therapy and enough Twelve Step meetings to know that shame is not a good thing to live with. Many of us, who grew up in dysfunctional homes, were shamed as children when we had no defenses. The "I'm not good enough" message is lodged deep within. It takes time and effort and help to let go of shame. And that's what I need to do now.

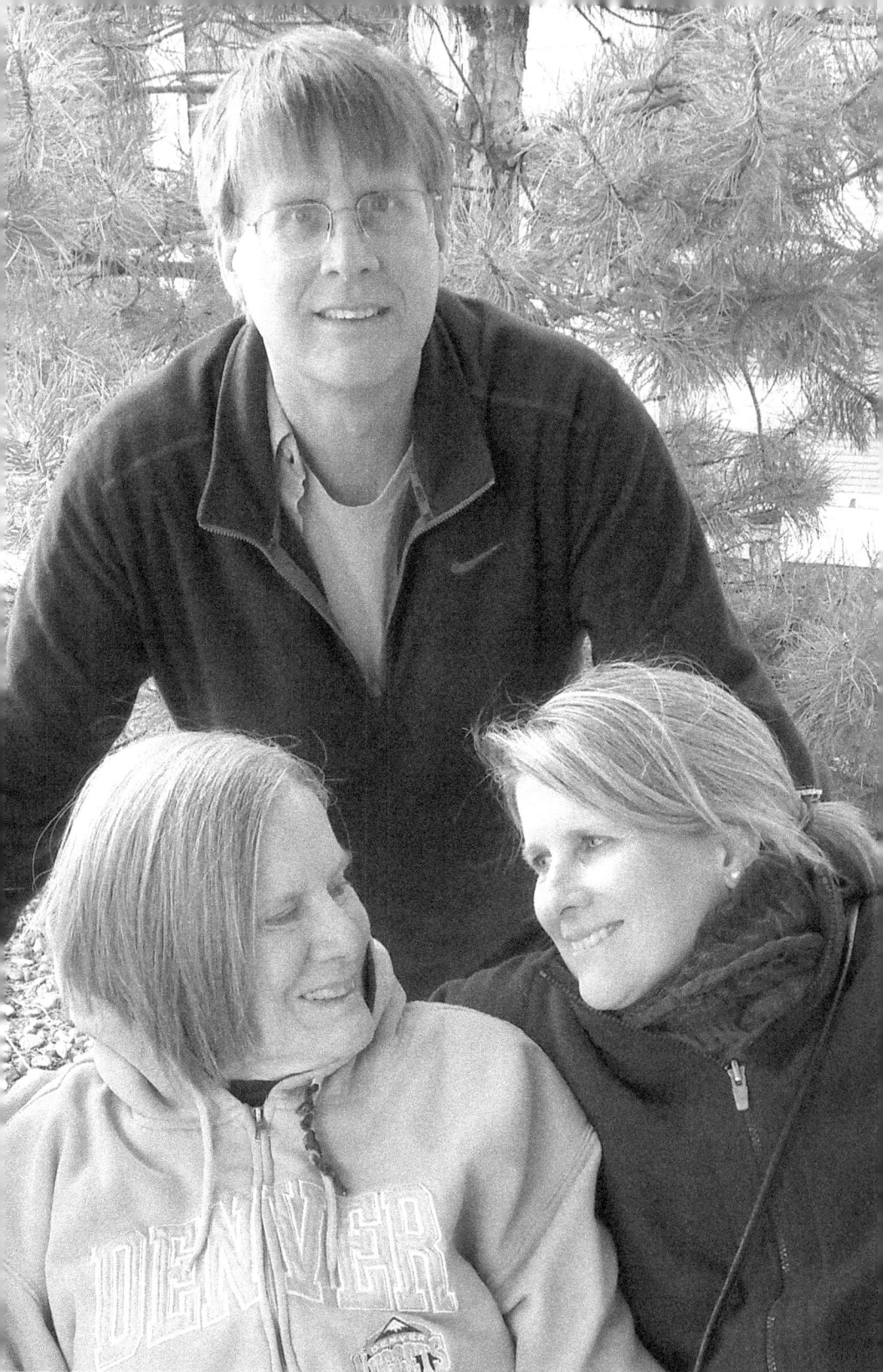

Molly outside memory-care facility with her son Chris and daughter Nora.

NORA'S PERMISSION

Alzheimer's affects the whole family, so the whole family needs to be involved in decisions about care. Sure, that's just common sense. I'll make every effort to include Molly's children. All of them: the three children Molly already had when we met and the three we adopted together from the Philippines.

It sounded simple and straightforward. But that was before I understood that this couldn't be one-size-fits-all. Each of Molly's children would react to their Mom's illness and decline in his or her own way, and I'd be jumping through hoops trying to keep everyone happy.

Luckily for me, her daughter Nora (third of the older kids) was easy. Nora's a doctor; she deals with illness all the time; she is level headed and warm hearted. She was always ready to say, "I really appreciate what you're doing for Mom." When she visited from New Orleans, I went with her and her brother Chris on a tour of the facility. Dr. Nora pronounced it a good place and agreed it was right for her Mom when the time came.

When the time did come, it really hit Nora hard: No denying or equivocating. Her Mom had an untreatable, terminal illness. On the phone, she told me how she was coping, "I clean, and then I cry. Then, I clean some more, and I cry." I cried, too.

On her next visit, Nora and I went together to pick up Molly and bring her to Chris's home for a Christmas tree trimming party. We all tried to pretend that it was just the same as last year, except that Molly had to go home early. Molly was somewhat disoriented and definitely incoherent when she spoke. No one commented on it, but we all understood that it was clearly not the same.

Later in the evening, when the grandkids went to the basement to play dodgeball, Molly, Chris, Nora, and I were left looking at the tree. The mood shifted and lightened. It brought back the time twenty-nine years earlier when Molly and I celebrated our first Christmas together and Chris and Nora were visiting. It felt right and good.

Other times while I was with Nora, I was strangely anxious. I kept telling her about the unit. "It's nice and small: it only houses fifty-two people."

"The staff is very well-trained. They're first rate." I repeated myself over and over compulsively.

On the way to the airport, just like in the last five minutes of a therapy session, I returned to the subject of the facility. And I realized what was happening: I wanted Nora's approval. I wanted her to tell me that it was a good place for her Mom. And, most importantly, that it was OK that I had put her there and not kept her at home longer.

"Nora, I can tell what's been going on with me over the past few days. I want your permission. I'm still feeling guilty about not keeping your Mom at home." "You can let go of that one," she said. "Thank you," I replied.

INCONTINENCE

I buy Depends by the case at Costco. You can imagine where this is going, so if you're going to be grossed out, you can turn the page.

In the dictionary, "incontinence" is such a beautifully euphemistic term. It's defined as "The quality or state of lacking normal voluntary control of excretory functions." The word comes from a proper Latin root meaning "to restrain."

I went to just enough workshops, lectures, and support group meetings to receive the consensus view on home care vs. institutional care. I was told by many experts and veterans that home care becomes difficult or impossible when the person wanders too much, behaves violently, or becomes incontinent.

At first, the whole issue of incontinence was part of my denial: if she's not peeing in the living room, then she's not too bad. But, of course, there did come a time when she peed on the carpet in the living room and pooped on the bedroom floor before she could get to the bathroom.

I kept telling myself that safety was the primary deciding factor about when she had to leave home, and I still believe it was first and foremost. However, incontinence did play a role.

After Molly went into the memory-care facility, her incontinence got worse quickly. She had a few "accidents" which the staff felt were unusual enough that they had to report them to me. It was evidence to them of how difficult she was to handle.

For about three weeks, I was not allowed to see Molly so she could become accustomed to the new routine and get used to someone else caring for her. When I did begin to visit, we developed a regular pattern, which included a walk to and around a nearby park. On these outings, I was responsible for Molly for an hour or more.

On a couple of occasions, I experienced total panic. Once we were in the park, and I pointed to the bright blue porta-potty near the tennis courts. Molly indicated she wanted to go there. When we got inside, I started undressing her and realized she had already pooped in her Depends.

There I am on my knees in front of her. I've just taken her shoes off so she's in her stocking feet. I'm pulling on her pant legs and she starts to pee, the urine puddling on the floor. I'm trying to move her so her socks won't get wet, and she's resisting me. I yell at her (absurdly), "Why are you doing this?" and I burst into tears.

I was "lacking normal voluntary control."

Now, I carry a spare Depends in my pocket whenever we go out. I have a lot more experience changing Molly. I don't panic anymore even when she resists being undressed. Living with Alzheimer's has forced me to redefine "normal."

PERFECTIONISM

I've told this on myself many times at Twelve Step meetings. When I was growing up, my Father expected me to be a genius (like everyone said he was); my Mother expected me to be a saint (like everyone said she was). When I was young, I thought it was harder to meet my Father's expectations: as I've gotten older, I've come to realize it's much harder to meet my Mother's expectations. I tell this to explain my character defect of perfectionism.

This behavior was reinforced by the magical thinking of a child. If I were really, really good, then Dad wouldn't yell at Mother because there were no clean t-shirts. He wouldn't smash the coffee pot on the kitchen floor or punch a hole in the wall in his rage. He wouldn't knock my little brother across the room with the back of his hand.

If I were really, really good, then Mother wouldn't be so depressed. Then we could all stop worrying about her going crazy and leaving us alone.

So I was really, really good: I was a straight-A student in school. I was an altar boy and so devout that some of the nuns picked me out as a candidate for the priesthood. I was a virgin until I went to college.

Of course, the magic didn't work. The real problems of alcoholism and depression remained, but somehow I still clung to the belief that being perfect is the way to live.

Since I'd been trying to be perfect for a long time, it wasn't surprising that when Molly was diagnosed with Alzheimer's, I was determined to be the perfect caregiver. I was never going to lose patience and yell at her in frustration. No, never. I was never going to let my guard down so she could wander miles away from home. No, never. I was never going to let my hurt feelings show when she hit me. No, never.

I did, in fact, get frustrated and distracted and hurt, but I had been so determined that it was hard to forgive myself. Part of me still wanted to be perfect, though by now I clearly understood that it was impossible.

Thus, my journey has included a growing acceptance of things as they are, not as they might be in some alternative, wished-for reality. In this life perfection is an illusion. Those who seem to be perfect in some way are invariably not. They only illustrate the saying, "Never judge a book by its cover."

Through caregiving, I've gradually learned a new perspective. The question is not "Am I doing it right?" but rather "Am I doing the best I can with the resources I have right now?" The honest answer is "Yes, I am doing the best I can."

SEX

In my book club at the public library, we were discussing Freud's theories about sex.

He based his hypotheses on the idea that attraction originates in two separate impulses. First, there is the "tenderness" associated with the infant's relationship with his or her mother and other family members. Second, there is the "sensual" (or erotic) impulse that begins with puberty. For Freud, these two must be harmoniously combined for the individual to have a healthy sex life.

Tenderness was always present between Molly and me. When she began to flirt with me in earnest, she sat next to me at a college event and stroked my hair. No erogenous zones were involved, but the effect was electric.

Not much later, we became lovers. There was no question that we found each other attractive and arousing.

All couples have their stories. This is one of ours: for our first anniversary, we wanted to do something special and romantic. We discovered that there was still an overnight train running up the East Coast to Montreal. We booked a sleeping compartment for the trip. We were both in the lower bunk naked making love when the train pulled into a station and stopped. But we couldn't stop. Afterwards, we laughed and hoped no one on the platform could see through the train windows. Almost having an audience actually added to the fun and excitement.

Alzheimer's affected our sexual relationship in several obvious ways. In one disconcerting episode Molly became obsessively sexual. She stimulated herself and wanted to be stimulated constantly. She was clearly frightened by the experience, perhaps because she was so unable to control her own body. Fortunately, this phase didn't last long.

A more fundamental change happened gradually. Molly and I ceased being partners as her needs and my responsibilities grew. I took over all the driving, all the cooking, all the laundry, all the telephone calls, all the mail. We became much more like parent and child every day.

As her cognitive abilities decreased, Molly also seemed to lose interest in sex. I wondered whether this might be temporary, but it wasn't. Molly was done. She really did seem to forget that her body could respond sexually. Perhaps she had regressed to a time before puberty when sex was not even a possibility.

Still the tenderness continues to this day. When Molly could no longer drive, she took it upon herself to massage my neck while I was driving, especially on longer trips. She often does that when we are together in the car.

And she strokes my hair.

EXHAUSTION AND SAFETY

"Will I ever get over the guilt?" I ask my psychiatrist. I'm talking about how I feel when I leave after visiting Molly. "Well, your feelings are your feelings," she says, "but you can tell yourself why she's where she is. You can remind yourself that she is safe and well cared for, in the best possible place. *And* she will forget." "After ten or twenty minutes, she won't remember?" I respond. "No, she won't."

Then, the doctor recommends author Byron Katie's techniques *(The Work)* for reframing my self-critical thoughts, "Katie's very cognitive and helpful." Later, my psychiatrist asks me, "Do you ever think about Molly's death?" "I used to quite a bit," I reply, "but now when I see her with all the other residents . . . She is physically one of the healthiest people in the place. Some of them are so frail: they can't walk; they can't eat; they can hardly speak. Molly has no heart trouble; she has no diabetes. I compare her to them, and I don't see her dying any time soon."

"What I think about now is the time when she won't recognize me. That seems like a more imminent thing that'll be really hard to take."

Knowing so little about how the disease progresses, including when certain abilities or functions will disappear, is confusing and frustrating. When we got the confirming/for-sure diagnosis—based on an MRI of Molly's brain that showed the tell-tale tangles—I did some research and asked questions of doctors. They were supposed to know something, but certainly they didn't know enough to satisfy my curiosity or calm my fears. "When you know an Alzheimer's patient, you know *one* Alzheimer's patient," one of the doctors said. "Each case is unique."

One of things I read (which later took on more and more significance) was that the average time from diagnosis to death for an Alzheimer's patient is eight to fifteen years. At first, I made assumptions based on the lower figure. A big assumption concerned when it would be time for Molly to leave home. If she was only going to live for eight years, I could probably wait five or six years to place her. By then, she would presumably be so out of it that she wouldn't notice the changes. Well, that sure didn't work out at all as I had imagined.

For one thing, I didn't count on my own limitations. At a certain point I would face burnout. Later safety would become a greater and greater concern as she got worse. At a certain point, I would have to admit that I could no longer keep her safe at home. I would have to sleep, take a shower, go to the bathroom. Who would watch Molly then? Who would keep her away from the stove and sharp objects?

I did get in-home respite care after four years on my own. That helped, but both my psychiatrist and my expert sister predicted that it wouldn't be enough, that I was still headed for total exhaustion. Exhaustion and unsafe conditions both arrived after about five years.

Molly was also much more anxious and disoriented, sometimes slipping into what looked like psychosis.

I had to face the fact that Molly's quality of life was often not good, despite my best efforts. I needed more help and more time off. She needed more care than any one or two people could give. The decision to move her to the memory-care unit was not easy, but it was necessary.

It was my own version of a Twelve Step slogan, "I can't; they can; guess I'll let them."

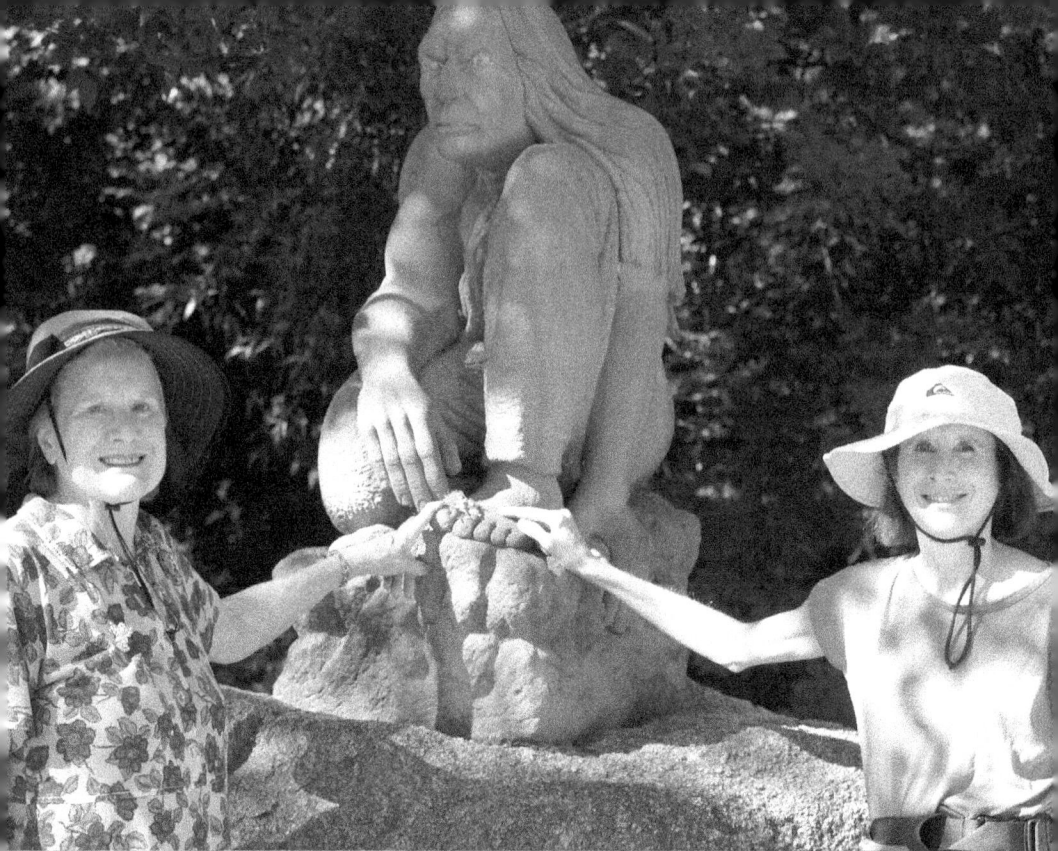
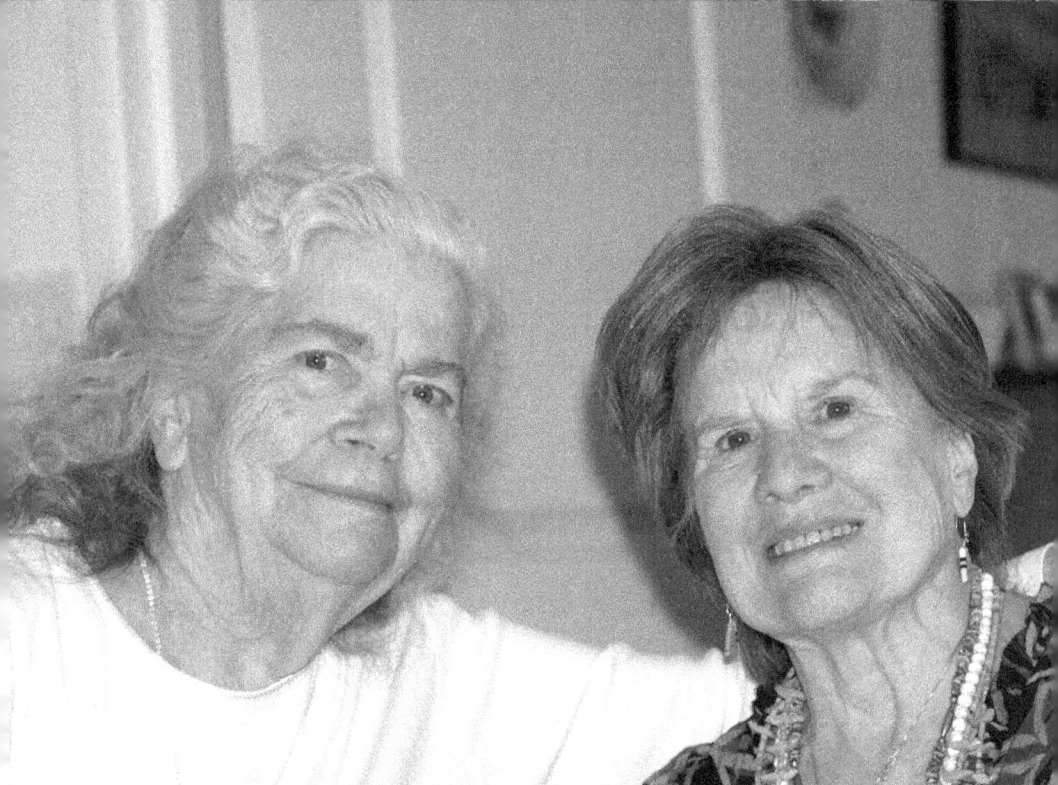

Molly and her daughter Cathy at the trailhead for the Boulder Creek Trail.
Molly and her mother-in-law Winifred in Chicago.

WANDERING AND ANGEL COIN

I have come to dislike, almost hate, single-sex restrooms. For a time, it seemed their only function was to give Molly the opportunity to wander.

After we moved down from the mountains to Boulder where Molly could breathe without extra oxygen, we got in the habit of walking the Boulder Creek Path almost every day. We followed a section of this walking, running, and biking path that began at the public library and followed the water for two and a half miles into the canyon.

One mile upstream from the library there is a park. In the park is a stone building with women's and men's restrooms. One day we got to the park, and Molly and I each went into a different side. I came out and waited for her. I waited a while and finally asked a woman going in if she would look for Molly inside. She reported that there was no one there.

I thought briefly about which way Molly was likely to have gone. She would probably be looking for me and would head further upstream. I started out to find her, my stomach tightening and my blood racing.

I passed people on the trail and asked, "Have you seen a woman with blonde hair and a blue jacket?" "Yes, she's up the trail, but we saw her ten minutes ago." Molly was then a strong walker: she was probably half a mile ahead of me, and I didn't know how I would ever catch up.

At about the two-mile mark, I was beginning to lose hope. I met a couple on the trail and explained about Molly's condition. They had indeed seen her, but past the end of the trail walking determinedly up the road with cars going by. They offered to drive me along the highway until we found her.

We did find her a couple of miles further along. Molly was walking straight ahead as though she had a goal in mind. She did not seem at all surprised to see me. She got into the car, and we gave her water. We all drove back to the library where Molly and I had parked our car. As I got out of the strangers' vehicle, I handed the driver a guardian angel coin I had been carrying in my pocket.

The coin was a gift from a different stranger after a previous walk. On that occasion Molly and I were at a market having coffee and pastries. We had just returned from a relatively long trek on a warm day. Molly's forehead was damp with sweat, so I reached over and mopped her brow. A man at the next table came over to us. "I see how you have been caring for your wife, and I want to give you this," he said. It was the guardian angel coin. "You may keep it as long as you like and pass it on when you wish."

I don't remember how many weeks I had that coin in my pocket, but when I passed it on, I knew it was at the right time and to the right person.

EATING

How will it be for Molly when the disease has progressed even further? The doctors and experts don't know for sure, but I have some idea. I can tell some things by observing the other residents in Molly's facility, most of whom are far more advanced than she.

I often sit with Molly at lunch. The residents have assigned tables and places, and Molly sits with others who need some help with eating. Molly is there because she spits out food she cannot chew or doesn't like the taste of. Anything that requires chewing, like a piece of chicken, must be cut into bite-sized chunks.

At first, there was concern that she wasn't getting enough calories to maintain her body weight. When she didn't consume what was offered, she was given a nutrition drink instead. Since I didn't like the sugar water product they were giving her I was able to find some health food smoothies that were both tasty and nutritious.

I also discovered one food that she never had any trouble with: chicken noodle soup. It's soft, and she always eats all of it. Now she has it for lunch every day. In fact, Molly is, in general, an eager and hearty eater. She will always eat soup and soft foods, like mashed potatoes. She is one of the few residents who has gained weight during her stay.

The other residents at Molly's table are much worse off. Some can't chew or swallow without difficulty, and some won't eat at all on a given day. Some require a care partner to put the food into their mouths for them. One woman falls asleep at the table and has to be awakened and fed. One man has recently turned down everything except dessert. I've also seen him take a second dessert from another resident when no one was looking. At least he knows what he wants.

Some people are physically disabled, including several who are wheelchair bound. Some just stare into space, their face muscles never moving. I see their physical decline day-by-day, month-by-month. It is very sad and frightening that someday Molly will be as helpless as some of her fellows are now.

So, a second question arises to go with "Why did this happen?" namely "What is left?" We humans are so used to communicating with words. A baby can talk at one and a half and express her needs. Molly cannot.

For a good long time, I thought Molly and I were communicating in the standard way, just with fewer words. Then I realized that the dialogue had often become a monologue. I would talk and ask questions. Molly would answer "Yes" to whatever I said.

It was a shock to recognize that there were times when she couldn't understand me anymore. I'm fine: I speak clearly and make sense. How could she not understand me?

This breakdown is not OK with me: it is frustrating and frightening, but it is part of the new normal. I will just have to live with it.

MY SIDE OF THE BED

I still sleep on my side of the bed. Not in the middle and certainly not on Molly's side.

When Molly and I were first together, I moved into her home. She had been divorced for a number of years. Her youngest daughter was away at college. Molly took in students as boarders to help with the rent, but it was her home, her place that she was sharing with me, and she had established her side of the bed.

We also adopted her habit for seating at the dining room table. Molly was accustomed to sitting at the head of the table. I wanted to be near her, not at the other end like rich people in movies. So I sat in the chair to her left. We could hold hands when we said grace. That's how we sat for twenty-nine years.

Now when I sit with Molly at lunch, I am usually to her right. I am close enough to help her cut up her food or use her napkin. Molly likes it if I am right next to her, our two chairs touching. If I come into the dining room and there is no chair available for me, Molly is confused and anxious. She expects me to sit next to her. That's how it has always been.

We lived in Molly's home until right before we got married. Then we bought a house, oddly enough, the first house that either of us had ever owned. That home was ours together.

One space we shared right from the beginning was the kitchen. Molly was a very good cook; her expertise included both fancy foods for Ivy League faculty dinners and mass quantities of ziti with tomato sauce to fill up growing children. I loved to cook with her and never ceased to marvel at how her soufflés always rose perfectly.

As an English professor, Molly needed a place to work at home: grading papers, writing articles, tutoring on-line. Wherever we lived, Molly had her special space. When we were designing our retirement home, what the architect intended as a breakfast nook became Molly's office.

Now her computer sits in a corner of our bedroom. She has not used it for a couple of years. At one point, she stopped reading her e-mail, and I did not know her password. I intend to recycle the machine somehow, but I wonder what is still on the C drive.

CELEBRATIONS

February 10, 2013

I'm no anthropologist, but it seems to be a basic human need to ritualize life with celebrations: marking holidays and anniversaries of birth, marriage, and other rites of passage. Celebrations are an opportunity for the tribe, clan, or family to gather and share.

In the twenty-first century, we're far away from the powerful intensity of a spring planting festival. Our survival doesn't depend on the colored eggs and chocolate rabbits in an Easter basket.

Why then do we still celebrate a birthday or an anniversary? There remains a strong desire to honor each other at regular intervals. I'm thinking about this today because it is our 29th wedding anniversary. This year we will not have a big family party. Molly certainly can't remember the wedding. She'd have no idea what an "anniversary" is or have any concept of how long twenty-nine years might be.

Part of our enduring desire for celebrations is that they are an opportunity to give and receive tokens of affection. Anyone who has ever gotten a hand-made birthday card from a child or grandchild knows. It is an opportunity to say "I love you, Dad."

"I love you, Grandma Molly."

I used to think quite differently. I was one of those skeptical people who thought the purpose of modern holidays was almost exclusively for commercial gain. After all, Mother's Day and Father's Day were inventions of card and flower and candy vendors. My perspective changed dramatically when Molly and I adopted our three children from another culture. In the Philippines, giving a gift, "ala ala," was very important. Our children hadn't had gifts before they came to America, and, more significantly, they had not been able to give gifts.

I asked our son Reynor how he knew that I was OK when we met. His life experience of adults would have left anyone unwilling to trust, especially to trust a stranger speaking an unknown language. He said, "Because you brought me ala ala." (It was a red toy pickup truck.)

Indeed, when the children went to school and were invited to friends' birthday parties, they were thrilled to pick out, wrap, and give ala ala themselves.

So, today, I will give Molly a pretty card on which I will write "I love you." We will go out to lunch together and share a special meal. It's important to celebrate whether Molly knows what it's all about or not. For I do.

SELF-CARE I

"Are you taking care of yourself?" my friends and family would begin.
"Well, I don't really know how to do that," I'd reply, "but I'm taking an art
class once a week." "That's good," they would say. It was most often a short
conversation that didn't get very far.

The simple truth was that I truly did not know how to take care of myself.
What I was good at was taking care of others. It's how I got positive
reinforcement. It's what made me a good person. I'd done it all my life and
always been praised for my kindness and generosity. What was this taking
care of myself stuff about all of a sudden?

I hadn't the foggiest notion of some of the basic principles of self-care. We
all need time and space to recharge when we are expending large amounts of
energy. We have weekends and vacations and holidays in the work world to
accomplish exactly that. Residents in an emergency room who work for
twenty-four hours straight or more are not much good until they rest. The
hospital had better give them a day off or face the consequences.

Caregiving has been described in one landmark book as *The Thirty-Six Hour
Day*. That's exactly what it often feels like. Under these circumstances, my
hour and a half of painting each week was a nice distraction, but it wasn't
going to do very much to restore my spent energy.

In the months since Molly has been in the memory-care unit, I have more
time and energy to take care of myself. Now I can see with twenty-twenty
hindsight things I wish I had known years ago. Now for me meditation
every morning is a key part of my life. For a few minutes I can let go of
anxiety and focus on breathing in and out. Such a simple thing, yet so
effective.

Before, when Molly was home, I would jump out of bed and begin breakfast.
I helped her get dressed. I got us out of the house so we could get our daily
exercise. I drove to the trail where we walked. This basic morning routine
took two hours or more. The thought of taking a few minutes to sit quietly
breathing in and out would never have occurred to me. There obviously
wasn't time for anything like that!

There's a consensus that hobbies and creative outlets are especially useful. That's why I always felt a positive response to the art lessons. These activities are good distractions, and they help release stress. Painting worked up to a point for me, but when I became overwhelmed, I just went dry. I didn't know how to paint the grief I felt when Molly could no longer read and write.

What I was doing on a regular basis was writing. I had joined a Fourth Step writing group (The AA/Al-Anon Fourth Step is "Made a searching and fearless moral inventory of ourselves.") where we were recording our lives incident by incident. Yet as a co-dependent and people pleaser, I couldn't bring myself to write about my life where anyone might see it and get mad at me. Now I write every day, and I am mostly beyond the fear that blocked me. I have found my outlet.

The other area in which I've had some success is lessening isolation. In the last year Molly was at home, I spent most of every day alone with her, and she couldn't carry on a conversation. On the days when the respite care person came, I would speak with the visitor for a few minutes when she arrived and when I returned. That might be it for the week. Not good. Now I am much better about contact with people. I made a rule for myself that I would have at least one adult conversation in person or on the phone every day. It really helps.

AFRAID OF VIOLENCE

February 15, 2013

Today, I am afraid. I had an email from one of the nurses at Molly's facility. "Early this week, Molly punched another resident's son in the face, without provocation . . . We've been noticing a decline in her patience with others, and she is quicker to strike out."

I didn't question the incident. Last week, she hit me in the face while I was undressing her in the restroom at a coffee shop.

Is this, indeed, a new phase in her decline? Is she becoming more violent as the cortex of her brain disintegrates? The very possibility, much less the reality, of this development is very disconcerting. It could have serious repercussions for her care, lead to more decisions I don't want to make right now or ever.

It also wreaks havoc with the story I have been telling myself and others. In it, Molly is an innocent victim of a terrible disease. The Universe or God is out to get her or me or both of us. There is no possible reason that she should suffer in this way. Molly has always been kind and generous and caring. She has been a wonderful mother and grandmother. She has been a great teacher for decades, always sensitive to the needs of her students and tireless in helping them learn and grow.

Even now, everyone in the unit likes her. The care partners are very fond of her. The other residents find her cheerful and pleasant.

Except when she's not. Except when she hits people in the face.

This is not a "good" story. It is not easy to tell. It makes me uncomfortable and scared. It shakes up my perspective big time.

I've encountered this kind of shakeup before in my Fourth Step writing. In writing our "searching and fearless moral inventory" for this step, we are asked to record all the events in our lives that we can remember. We are then asked to record separately our thoughts about the events and our feelings about them.

After a while, it becomes painfully obvious that many of the stories we told ourselves about our lives are just not true. Our thinking and feelings distorted the "facts." We thought we were being honest, but we often didn't recognize reality.

One of my untrue stories explained parts of my life with the statement "I was shy." What is true is that I was socially isolated as a child and an adolescent. My father was an alcoholic and an abuser; my mother was depressed; we had too many children (fourteen); we were very poor. We kept to ourselves and maintained our secrets. I never invited friends to the house. I had a grand total of three dates in high school, one of which was to a Sadie Hawkins dance where the girl asked me.

I was convinced I was born with a shy gene, that shyness was a permanent part of my personality and my behavior. That's what I told people about myself until I was past forty.

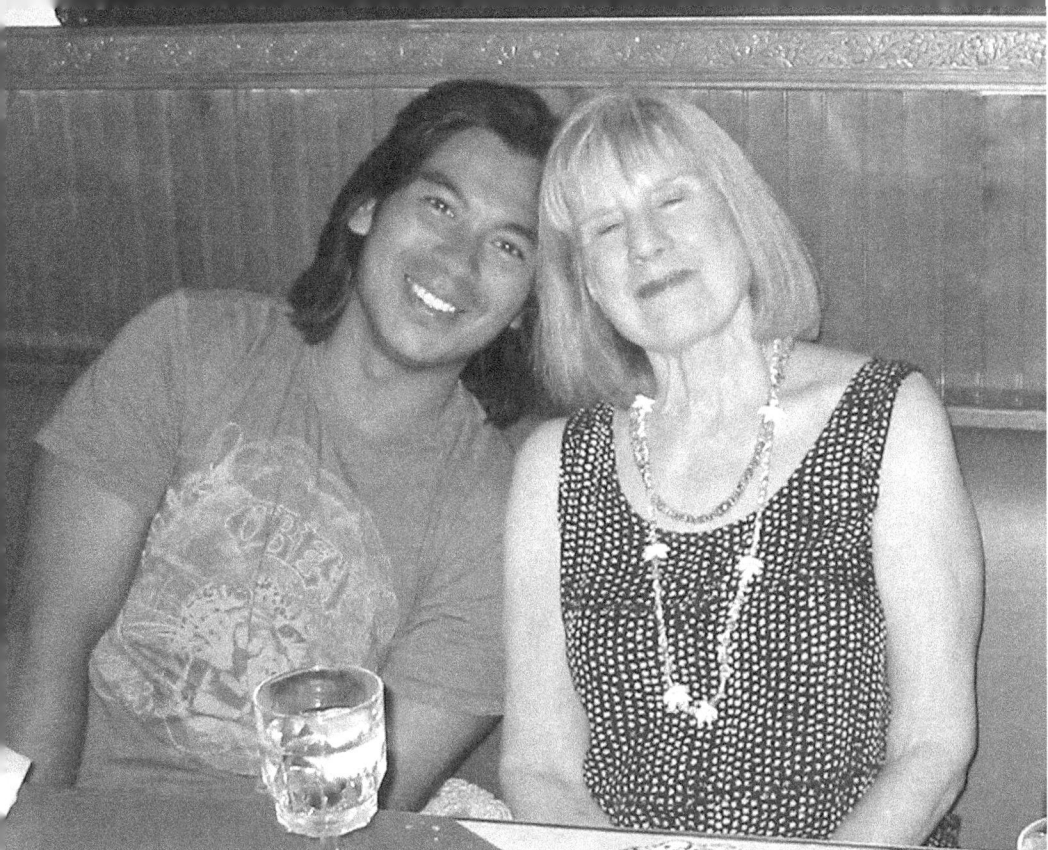

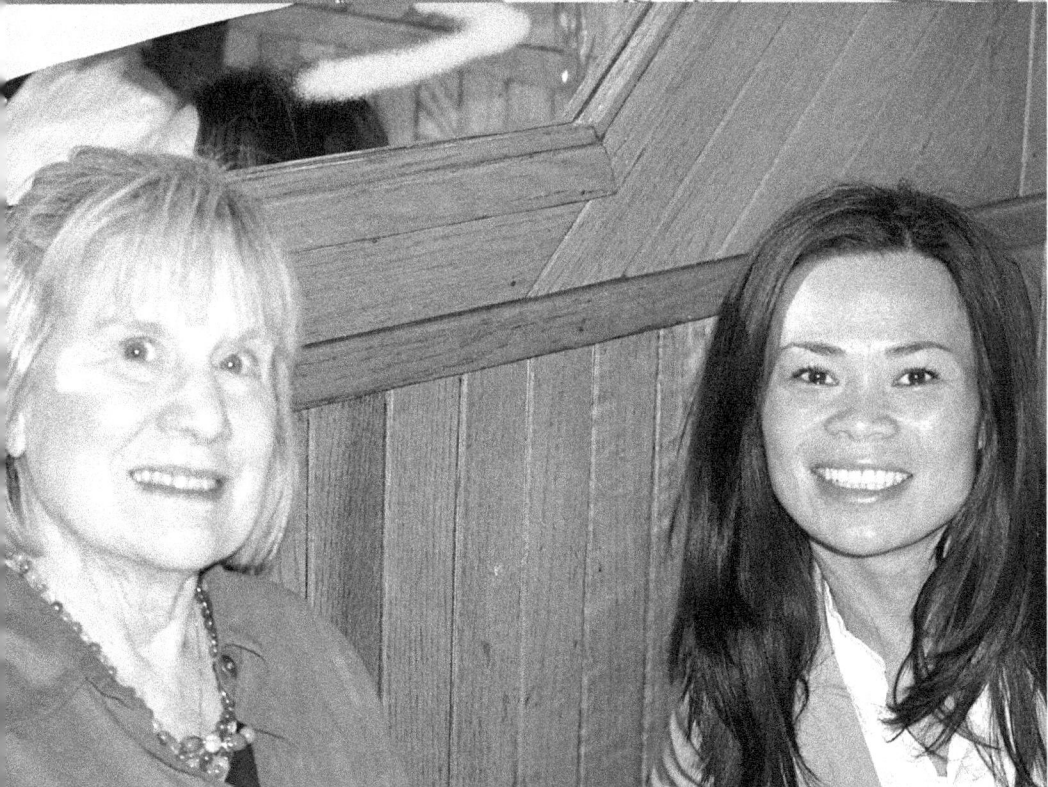

Molly with son Reynor in Hawaii 2007.
Molly with daughter Mae in Brooklyn, NY.

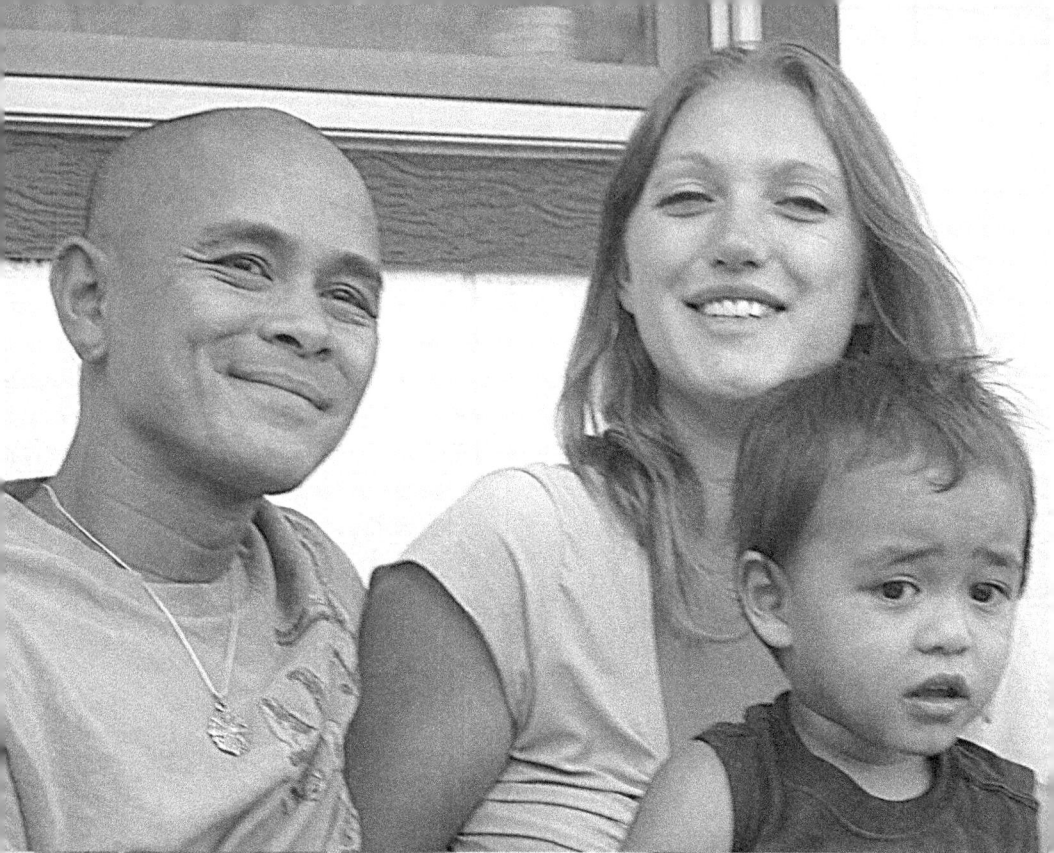

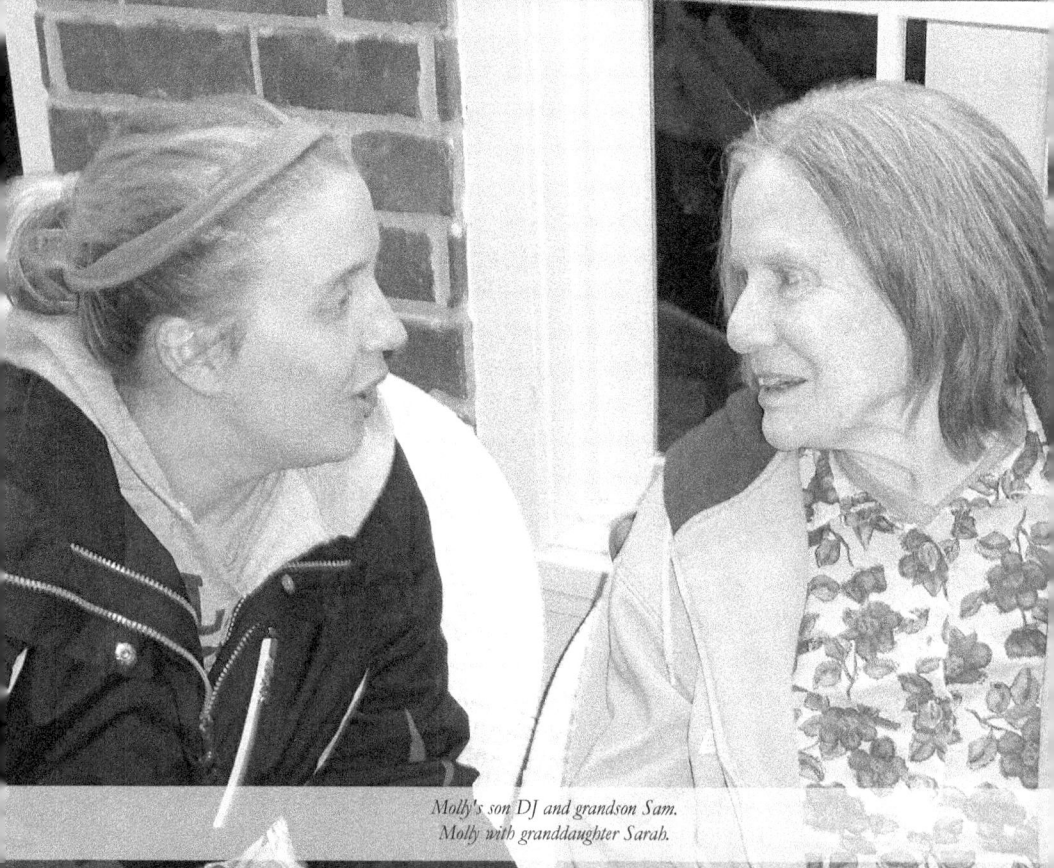

Molly's son DJ and grandson Sam.
Molly with granddaughter Sarah.

But it's not true. I am not shy: I was ashamed as a child because I was hiding the family's dark secrets. I have been an actor, a professor, and a teacher of public speaking. I greet strangers on the elevator and talk about the weather or sports. The shyness story was just plain false.

Now I have to figure out what to think and say about Molly. Our reality just got more complicated. I need to change the story I tell myself and others about Molly. In the old version, Molly was always kind and gentle. Now Molly has a disease that has destroyed parts of her brain, and she may hit someone.

IT'S THE DISEASE

(At the Great Books Club at the Public Library)
FRIEND: How is Molly doing?
WILLEM: She's doing all right, but she's gotten more aggressive. She's been hitting and kicking people this week, so they're upping her meds. And it's hard for me, because Molly is not an aggressive person.
FRIEND: You're right. Molly is the sweetest. (Pause) Well, are they telling you that it's the disease not Molly?
WILLEM: No, that's my job.

Indeed, I'm the one who needs to tell myself that Molly's behavior is because of Alzheimer's. I know it's my job because of my years in Twelve Step programs. Alcoholism is a disease. How alcoholics behave depends on how sick they are.

At our Al-Anon meetings and in our literature, we learn to separate the disease from the person. The *Hope for Today* volume of daily readings includes this entry, "Learning more about the disease of alcoholism as a disease taught me that my father wasn't a bad person. He was a person with a disease that made him do bad things."

This insight is key to getting out of the habits of blame and resentment towards the alcoholic. As long as we family members let those habits control us, we cannot get better ourselves. I've worked on letting go of blame and resentment for over twenty years.

Today, I need to remind myself that Molly's Alzheimer's is similar to alcoholism. When Molly's respite caregiver first told me that Molly had hit her and kicked her, I just couldn't believe it. Molly must have just been shooing her away. She wouldn't actually attack anyone. That's just not like Molly, Molly the person I know and love.

Indeed, it's not Molly. Molly's surprising behavior is just her Alzheimer's disease coming out.

WOULD YOU STILL LOVE ME?

Our adopted children often tested limits. Would we come looking for them if they ran away? Yes, we would. Would we still care for them if they tore apart a gift we had given them? Yes, we would. Would we still love them if they hit us? More challenging, but, yes, we would.

Once while we were on a long car trip, they made a game out of it. They would make the most grotesque faces they could and ask, "Would you still take me if I looked like this?" It made us all laugh. Yet as Freud said, "There are no jokes." They really wanted to know how much we wanted them and how much we loved them.

Whether they understood what they were asking or not, they wanted to know if our love was unconditional. As little children, I believe they experienced family love, but then their biological mother died and their father left to start a new family with another woman. So, for them, family love couldn't be trusted. How were they to know that we strangers would not abandon them, too? They had to keep asking and testing, because they couldn't be sure.

I believe Molly has similar questions now. "Will you still love me if I cannot remember your name?" "Yes, I will." But love in what way? It must be different now, mustn't it?

Almost every time I visit, Molly says, "I love you, and I want to be with you. Forever." This is a pretty good definition of love: being in the presence of the person you care about. "I want to be with you, my love. When we are together, I experience joy. And when we are apart, I long for us to be together again."

I have several views on love. One is a romantic's notion. Each of us is incomplete without our soulmate. When we come together, we are whole and we enjoy bliss in that union. We experience life as parts of one person.

Another of my views defines a loving relationship as a partnership of equals. When we love someone, we admire and cherish the gifts each has to offer. Also we accept our differences as less important than what we share.

Molly today is not the same as the woman I fell in love with and spent the last three decades with. How do I love her now? It can't be as simple as imagining her ten years ago and loving that person though I believe that does play a role.

As with adopting our children, marrying Molly was a commitment to unconditional love. The commitment stands even under the conditions of Alzheimer's, when we are no longer equal partners and we no longer experience life with and through each other.

When Molly says, "I love you," I say, "I love you" back. I mean what I say, even though I don't—and perhaps never can—fully understand what love is for us now.

TRAVEL WHILE YOU CAN

February 20, 2013

When it became clear that soon Molly would not be able to travel, I made the decision to take some trips while she still could. She was still nearly fluent in Italian, especially the first time we went together.

Years earlier, we had taken a wonderful trip to Great Britain as our pre-wedding honeymoon. We were teaching at a college that offered study trips to students during the break between semesters. The year we got married, Molly and I hosted the trip to England and Scotland, focusing on drama. We went to Stratford and saw Shakespeare's *Measure for Measure*. We saw plays in London and Edinburgh. We had class discussions before and after each performance, and the students wrote papers on the plays.

After thirteen days herding nineteen students, we took them to the airport and waved good-bye. Now we were free to enjoy each other, which we did on a trip to Cornwall, where ocean currents keep it warm in winter and the gardens are in bloom in February.

That was the beginning of many trips. Molly often delivered academic papers at international conferences in the summer so we had opportunities to go all over Europe.

About three and a half years ago when I realized that Molly was becoming much more confused and disoriented by unfamiliar places and situations, I planned our last big trip. We would return to Italy one more time.

It went remarkably well. I was with Molly every minute, and she did not have the itch to wander. I did the driving and the map reading. She appreciated the exquisite art and the sacred sites connected to St. Francis of Assisi and St. Benedict. It was extraordinarily moving to see St. Francis's cloak and sandals and a letter he had written 900 years ago.

At Christmas this year, I traveled solo to visit family in California. It was terribly strange to leave Molly behind. She wasn't in front of me in the security line at the airport. She wasn't sitting next to me on the plane. She wasn't there when my sister hugged me.

Today, I am flying east to see our newest grandchild, who is two weeks old. I am alone on the plane, sitting next to strangers. It does not feel right.

I have brought along photos of Molly to share with our daughter and son-in-law and old friends. It is one way to bring Molly with me. However when I take pictures of baby Sophia, Molly will not be in them. It is not fair. I do not think I will ever get used to it.

OLD FRIENDS

On my trip to the East Coast I spent the evening with very old friends of Molly, Alicia and Jerry, a couple who knew her almost twenty years before I did. We had seen them about a year and a half ago when Molly was still able to travel.

They wanted to know how she was doing. "What is her mood like? "Does she have any friends there?" "What does she do when you are not around?"

I answered as best I could. "She is OK. She smiles and laughs. We skip down the sidewalk together when we go out."

"When she first got there, she latched onto all the men—residents and staff-and called them all 'Papa,' which is the name the grandchildren use for me. Then for a while she hung out with a woman named Pat, but Pat has declined and spends most of her time sleeping now. There is a guy she sits with sometimes who wears a Navy baseball cap. I don't know his name, but I'll have to find out what it is."

"I watched parts of a couple of movies with her and sang along with the songs she knew. One was *Carousel,* which has the wonderful song 'If I Loved You' right at the beginning." "I know that song," Alicia said, and we sang together "If I loved you, time and again I would try to say all I'd want you to know. If I loved you, words wouldn't come in an easy way, round in circles I'd go . . ."

Words are not at all easy for Molly now, but when they are attached to a melody, she remembers them. With Alzheimer's music is one of the last things to go.

I described to her friends how much Molly still enjoys the music in her life, singing along with the performers who come on Monday, Wednesday, and Friday, as well as singing the hymns at the Sunday service.

I showed Alicia and Jerry recent photographs of Molly—Molly at the fall dance, Molly at the Christmas party, Molly at Chris's house. They were reassured, "She looks just the same." They want that to be true: that she looks the same and is the same. That she has the same spirit, the same sense of humor, the same ways of being the Molly they know and love.

I am well aware that she is not the same. I know they would be shocked to see her spill her food down the front of her clothes, shocked to see her "get lost" two blocks from where she lives, shocked to see her wet herself at the coffee shop.

I do not say any of these things out loud. Denial can be lovely when it works. Actually I can see the good in happy memories of better days with the Molly that was.

I like to go there sometimes myself. It can be a wonderful place.

WHY IS GRANDMA MOLLY SICK?

Our three-year-old grandson asked, "Why did Grandma Molly get sick?" "The doctors don't know, and I don't know either," I had to say.

That is certainly one of the frustrating things about Alzheimer's: there is no known cause that has been confirmed through research. There is, of course, research that points to a damaged gene that increases the hereditary risk, but that does not account for the large majority of the over 5 million current cases.

Not knowing the cause directly affects the possibility of treatment. When we know the cause of disease with other major organs, we can develop treatments, including medications that address those causes and can cure the disease. Think heart disease or kidney disease or lung disease. They are often treatable, not least because medical science has determined their causes.

Alzheimer's is different. We know about the plaque and the tangles in the nervous system of the brain, but we still do not know how and why these abnormalities develop. Now all the best available medications can do is slow down the degeneration, but they cannot in any way reverse the damage and regenerate healthy nerve bundles.

It is very frustrating for all involved (three-years-old or sixty-three) that we don't know why Grandma got sick, especially since Molly's parents exhibited no signs of dementia into their nineties.

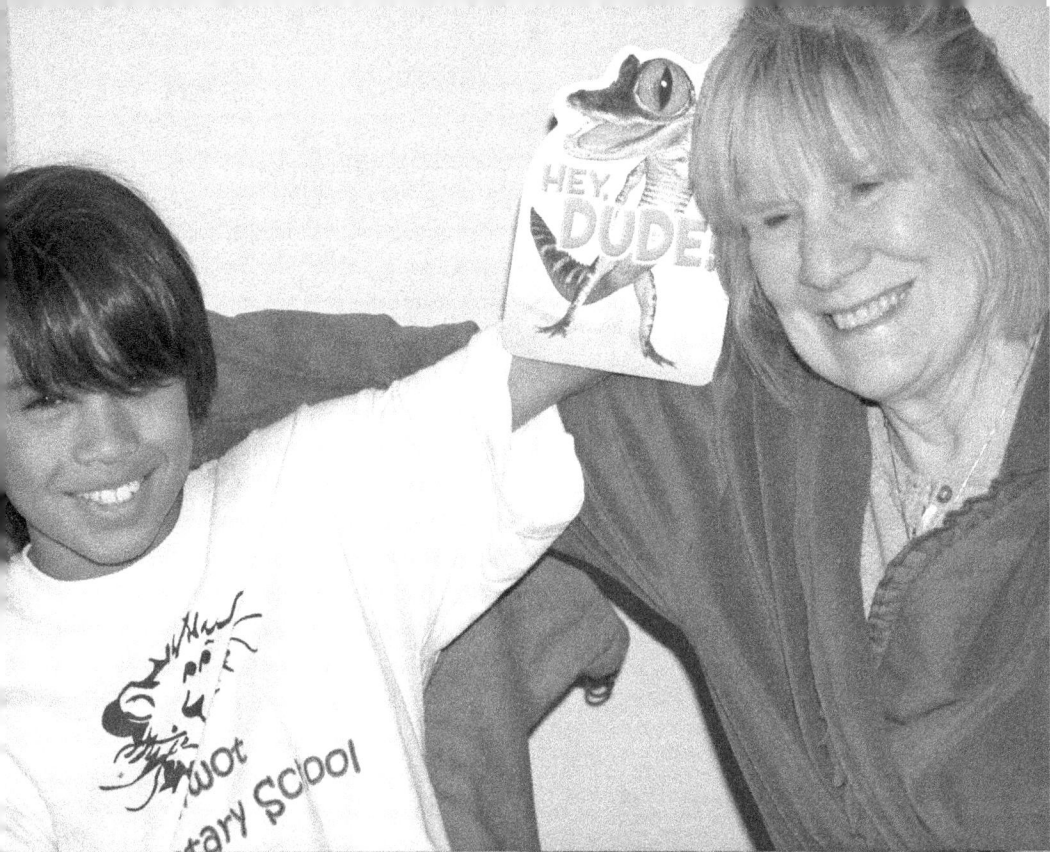

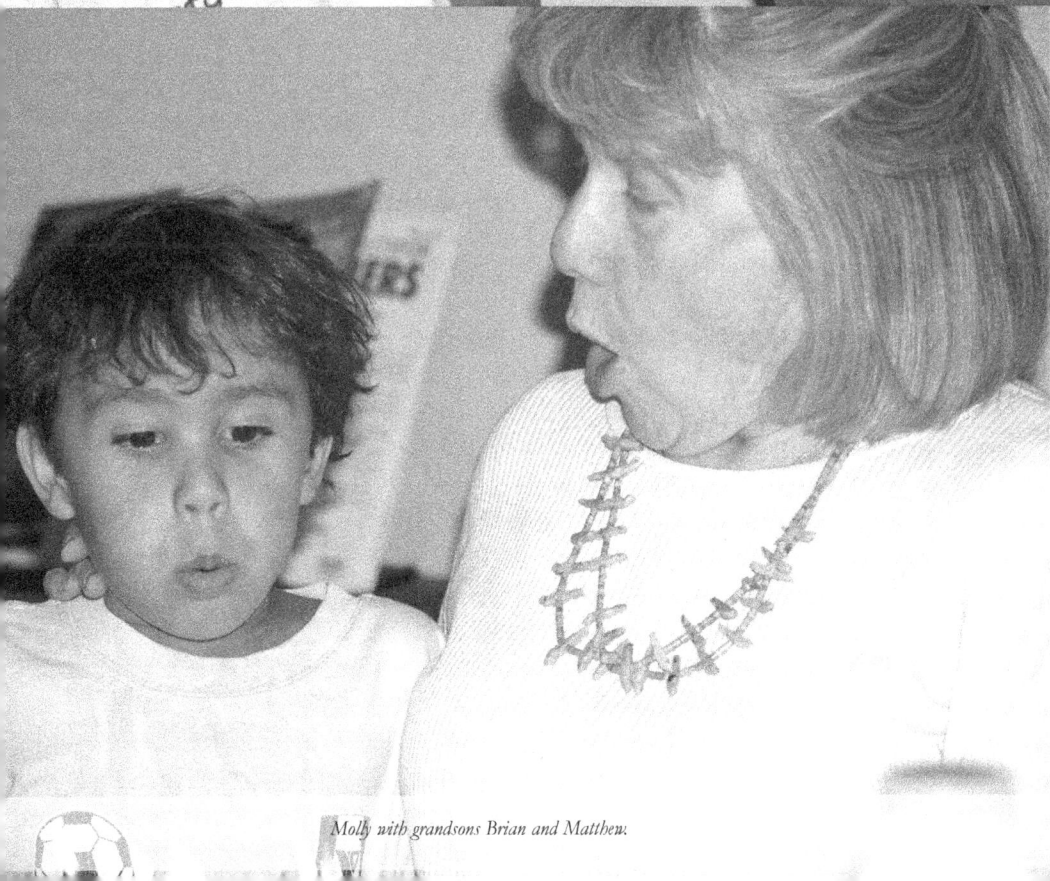

Molly with grandsons Brian and Matthew.

Absent the clear pattern of hereditary risk, the diagnosis almost always comes as a shock to both doctor and patient. "Doctor, I'm healthy; I exercise; I don't smoke or drink; I just lose my car keys and can't remember phone numbers." "Well that may be caused by stress or just be a normal part of aging." However, this time it isn't normal anything: it is Alzheimer's, a deadly and untreatable disease.

Molly and I were certainly shocked. She had no clue from her family history and no friends her age who had developed Alzheimer's. In many ways her brain seemed her strongest organ. Even after retirement, she continued teaching English part-time and did online tutoring for graduate students in nursing. She read theology and philosophy in our book club. She studied cultural anthropology, a whole new field for her, and wrote a brilliant paper on Afghan woman and wearing the burkha long before this issue appeared in the general media. How were we to know?

We had a moment of morbid curiosity when we read about aluminum poisoning from soda cans. Did drinking all those diet cokes cause the disease? Almost certainly not.

Still, I suspect that there is some pollutant in the environment now that wasn't there back in the days, back when Granny got senile just because she was getting old. There's got to be a cause, a reason for Alzheimer's. It can't just be random. Or can it?

WANDERING AND THE ANGEL SARAH

"I have always depended on the kindness of strangers." So says the character Blanche in the play *A Streetcar Named Desire* by Tennessee Williams.

I myself have relied on strangers to help me find Molly when she wandered. Many of the strangers were in uniform: police officers from the city and the county. They were remarkably helpful and successful, never seeming to resent the time and person-power devoted to one woman's safety.

A particularly memorable civilian helper was a woman named Sarah (or perhaps Sara). She told me her first name in the parking lot of the restaurant where Molly disappeared. She overheard me explaining that Molly had Alzheimer's when I asked if anyone had seen Molly after she came out of the women's restroom. One of the cooks had, indeed, seen her go out the back door.

Sarah volunteered to join in the search. "I have some time today so I'll go looking, too." She headed north and west while I went north and east. We met back in the parking lot about twenty minutes later. "No one has seen her in the stores between here and Pearl Street," she reported. I had not found her either. By then a critical mass of city police had arrived and started their own search. I started to cry, and Sarah held me.

A short time later, the police received a call from the police station located in the opposite direction of our searching. Molly had been found across the street from the station itself. Sarah and I hugged good-bye before I left to pick Molly up. I had never seen Sarah before and, most likely, will never see her again. Sarah was an angel who appeared at just the right moment and disappeared without a trace. Was she real or did I conjure her up out of my need?

After that incident, the police insisted that Molly wear a tracking device around her ankle. Molly hated it and tried to take it off and to get me to cut it off. I felt better thinking she would be traceable.

Unfortunately, we had occasions to test the technology, and it failed twice. One time, Molly was outside its range; the other time, it just wasn't working. The good news is that both times the police and EMTs were able to find Molly even without the device.

The last time Molly "escaped" I had just arrived home, and the respite caregiver told me Molly had gotten past her and out the door. We went in opposite directions, and I spotted Molly going around a corner down the block. I caught up to her. She did not seem surprised to see me and followed me willingly back home. She had just gotten the itch to move, to go somewhere, anywhere.

I never knew when Molly's urge to wander was going to happen although I was most often asleep when she took off. Maybe she thought I would stop her if I were awake?

I also installed a special device high on the door that blocked her opening it. That did the trick for any time we were at home. Also I got completely bold about declaring every restroom a "family restroom" where I could be with her all the time.

WISDOM OF FORGETTING

In many cultures people look to their elders for wisdom. It seems like common sense: those who have already experienced life know more about it than those who have yet to experience life.

Before her illness took hold, Molly exhibited that kind of wisdom. She had certainly experienced life. She had watched her parents go through all of the stages from young adulthood to fragile old age. She had raised three children and then raised three more children. She had been a pioneer in her career, the third woman to receive a Ph.D. in English from Princeton. She had lived through an especially tumultuous time in American society, including the civil rights movement, the women's movement, the gay rights movement, and too many wars from World War II to Iraq.

In her professional life as an English professor, she was accorded the respect due an elder stateswoman. Younger colleagues came to her for advice. Students modeled themselves on her. Even administrators looked to her for leadership.

All of that was before Alzheimer's. What about now? Might she still have something to teach us about life? Is she modeling anything from which we might benefit?

I tend to think of Alzheimer's in terms of what she can't do. After all, her diagnosis included an MRI that literally showed brain damage. In particular she can't remember.

Yet from another point of view that means she *can* forget. If I had asked Molly the question, "What has happened in your life that you would like to forget?" I believe I know what she would have answered. "I'd like to forget Kevin's death." Molly lost Kevin, who would have been her second child, when he was a couple of months old. She grieved for him for decades, especially on the anniversary of his passing.

There is a whole branch of psychotherapy dedicated to releasing the pain of the past and anxiety about the future. In Melody Beattie's book *The Language of Letting Go*, the index lists twenty-three things a recovering person might want to let go of, from anger to worry.

Molly no longer needs such therapy. Our friend Beth says Molly has achieved peace and contentment because she is always in the present moment. She does not regret the past nor worry about the future. Her only concern is what is happening right now.

No one need ever tell Molly to "stop and smell the roses." She always takes innocent pleasure in simple things: the blue sky on a sunny day, the feel of ice cream on her tongue, the melody of a beautiful song, the familiar events in a favorite story.

There is wisdom in this state of grace. I have to do a lot of meditating to get beyond thoughts of the past and future, and being fully in the present may only last for a few seconds. Molly is always there.

ADULT-CHILD

I remember well a popular movement in self-help psychology called transactional analysis, or TA. It was widely disseminated in such best selling books as *I'm OK, You're OK* and *Games People Play*. In TA theory, people have three basic modes of behavior, as a parent, as an adult, or as a child. Even between adults, there could be situations where effective interaction involved parent-to-child and child-to-parent communication. But most often the best interactions, and certainly the best lasting relationships, were when two individuals communicated as adult to adult.

I read these books, and I thought they demonstrated common sense. In particular, if either Molly or I treated the other as a parent would treat a child, instead of how an adult would relate to an adult, things would not work out very well. In TA terms, adult-to-adult was right for Molly and me.

But is it still the appropriate behavior now? Over the course of her decline, I took on more and more parent-like responsibility for Molly's wellbeing and safety. I did the cooking when she could no longer handle the stove. I did the driving and paid the bills and made the appointments and gave her medications. It was easy to see our new relationship as parent-child.

This was reinforced by some of Molly's behavior. Yesterday I saw her sticking out her tongue at another resident, something she has probably not done since she was a child. She resists having her hair washed, much like her granddaughter did at age two. Like a child, she cries very easily when she is upset by small things.

Inevitably I will feel and act like a parent to Molly, especially when I am trying to keep her safe. When we cross the street, I must interpret the signals and watch for turning cars. She cannot do this for herself. So I hold her hand and tell her when to cross and when to wait.

The challenge then is to give Molly opportunities to make choices: she is not helpless and she does have her own opinions and her own desires. Yesterday, I took her to a place where we have walked together hundreds of times over the years. It is a path along the creek that starts at the public library.

After we parked, I asked Molly if she would like to take a walk. She said, "Yes," and I proceeded to head upstream on our customary route. But she pointed the other way. So this time we went downstream towards the city park. Every time we came to a crossroads, she pointed the way and I followed her lead. She seemed happy to be in charge for once.

As we walked, I was reminded of one of the slogans I learned in my 12 step program, "How important is it?" The answer most often is "Not very." If it is not unsafe, Molly gets to decide. She likes that. For a few minutes, I can relax and let go of parental responsibility. I may even get to relive the joyful feeling of being a child.

DEATH, FINAL TABOO SUBJECT

I was talking to a friend after seeing the film *Quartet*, which depicts elderly musicians in a retirement home in England. She said seeing the old people on the screen made her think about how close she herself is to the end of life.

I opined, "Seeing the residents at Molly's place—how frail they are, how confused—makes me think the opposite. I'm still a long way from that state. I've got lots of good years left."

And, I've been telling myself and everyone else, so does Molly. I always point out that she is physically active, that she has no heart disease or diabetes. I say that she may live a long time. I quote what I read about the average span from diagnosis with Alzheimer's to death being from "eight to fifteen years." By that standard, she may well have ten years left (or more). After all, it is an "average."

Of course, no one knows for sure. What is true is that Molly has an incurable, terminal disease. She may yet die of a surprise heart attack, but, failing such an event, she will die from the effects of Alzheimer's. As I understand it, the brain eventually forgets everything, including telling the lungs to breathe and the heart to beat.

This is not something I want to think about. I admit to being in denial. I am emphatically far away from acceptance. Isn't it bad enough that Molly can't write her name? Can't remember what she had for lunch ten minutes later? Can't control her bladder?

Death. That's really bad, really final.

I don't accept it as a real and, perhaps, near-term possibility. At least now, I can visit Molly every day. I can feel her hand in mine, hear her voice when we sing, watch her eyes light up when she smiles. I can enjoy our time together now, and I can use her presence to remember all the things we shared over the years.

What happens when she's really, completely gone? I know. I know. She will always be in my heart and in my mind. I will still have wonderful memories of her, but it will not be the same. It will be lonelier.

It is sad even to think of it. Someday I will have to face it, even accept it.

No. Not now. Not yet. She is still here. Thank God.

A LOVING GOD?

After Molly went into the memory-care unit, I had a real sense that my life was over, that it had lost its purpose. I didn't see any way forward.

I thought the stars had aligned against us in a profound way. Molly and I were good people. We made some mistakes, but, on the whole, we did most everything right. We loved each other. We adopted our three kids and raised them with the love they never had before they came to us. We worked hard. We especially cared about our students and made every effort to help them. I was even an honest real estate broker (I don't recommend it if you want to make a living).

So why all the bad stuff: my cancer, Molly's Alzheimer's, our son D.J.'s mental illness?

What seemed clear is that a loving God couldn't be involved. There were only two possibilities: either God was distant and didn't care, or God just didn't exist. I vacillated between the two positions, but mostly I was plain angry with God.

I talked about this in my Twelve Step meetings, and my sponsor had a suggestion. He and his wife had taken A Course in Miracles (ACIM). He explained that in the Course one learned about a God of Love. One also learned that our pain and suffering, indeed, the body and the whole physical world were but illusions. God held us in the love in which he created us, and our eternal selves were destined to be reunited with our Creator in Love and Light.

For whatever reason, the idea of being with people who believed in a God of Love seemed appealing, and I signed up for the Course.

A Course in Miracles has led to a major shift in my perspective. Now I can at least see the possibility that the following is true: Molly's Alzheimer's affects only her body, which is a material shell for her true spiritual self. Her true self is all right. God is taking care of her, and she will be peaceful and joyful with God in eternity.

I certainly want to believe that this is true. It is much better than where I started. It also lets me off the hook. If Molly's disease is meaningless compared to her spiritual life, then what I did or didn't do for her didn't matter. God is in charge, and God is taking good care of her. I don't have to worry or feel guilty.

I also have a new network of support in the Course in Miracles group. An interesting mix, we talk about philosophy and theology, about various forms of healing: physical, emotional, psychological, and spiritual and about spiritual experiences; insights; and small, everyday miracles.

The Course experience has proved to be cathartic, comforting, and stimulating. My original purpose in joining the group turns out to be true: it is good for me to be around people who believe in a God of Love.

B.J.

I am at the fall dance in November at the memory-care facility. It is my first experience of the wider community of residents and families all in one place at the same time. The mood is remarkably upbeat. These people really do know how to party.

Including Molly. I expect that she will want to rest between dances. No way: once she gets going, she wants to keep moving. The music is good, a singer using big band arrangements on CD. So we dance and dance some more.

I'm also interested in meeting people. I'm still pretty new to the whole thing. My expert sister Bernadette says that I will become part of the community and get to know these people well as time passes.

Molly doesn't give me much opportunity to talk to people, but there is one person I have to meet. Her name is B.J., and she has some of the most beautiful eyes I have ever seen. At one point, I am directly across the room from her and her family members.

I cross over to her and speak to the daughter "I have to meet your Mother because she has the most beautiful eyes." "Hello, I'm Mary, this is B.J. and this is B.J.'s grandson." I shift focus to the boy and we talk soccer for a few moments. Then I come back to B.J. and repeat the compliment about her eyes. She gives me a devastating smile, and we're friends on the spot.

B.J.'s most frequent visitor is Sally, her middle daughter. I have noticed that B.J. is slowing down, but I am still shocked when Sally tells me that B.J. is eighty-eight years old.

Sally and I send e-mails back and forth. Sally: *The hardest part is constantly learning to appreciate the person she is now. Sometimes I pretend that she is just a nice happy lady I visit, then I am not hurt and disappointed that she doesn't know things about me. Appreciating daily her laugh!* Willem: *I am in the great place that she is just a nice happy lady for me to visit.*

In the dining room the residents are carefully grouped together. Sometimes for the convenience of the staff, but also to acknowledge friendships that have developed. B.J. sits at the head of a table on the opposite side of the room from where Molly sits with the problem eaters.

My usual routine is to arrive during lunch and sit with Molly. Then we go to Molly's room and prepare to go out for a walk. As Molly and I head down the hall, we pass by B.J.'s table, and I quickly get in the habit of stopping by to greet her and her table mates and discuss the food of the day, the weather, etc.

B.J. always makes eye contact and smiles. Usually, she'll offer me some of her food. She is tiny and, I imagine, doesn't eat much, but like everyone else she loves sweets, especially ice cream. I sometimes take a bite of whatever is on offer, but she doesn't share her ice cream!

B.J. always sits in the first row for the musical guests. The other day, Molly and I returned from a walk a few minutes before the musician arrived. Everyone was already seated waiting, with B.J. right near the front door. "What's going on?" I asked her. "Not much."

Molly and I had been singing on our walk so I launched into "When you wore a tulip" for B.J. and the others. B.J. grinned, and I grinned back.

B.J.'s beautiful eyes are at their best when she smiles.

LESSONS LEARNED

A friend asked, "In this process with Molly, what have you learned?" Such a simple and obvious question, but this is the first time anyone has asked it directly.

I paused, and what popped into my mind was patience. As we go through life with work and children, we get used to scheduling—often down to the minute. If I have to be at work at 8:30, I have to catch the 7:35 train, which means I have to leave the house at 7:15, which means I set the alarm for 6:15. Life according to the clock.

Parents with small children know that real life, in fact, rarely if ever runs this way. I have had to learn that with Alzheimer's things take as long as they take. I said to my friend, "If you expect something to take an hour and it winds up taking two hours and you spend the second hour saying to yourself 'This is terrible. We are going to be late. Why is it taking so long?' you will quickly drive yourself crazy." So one of the things I have learned is patience, which in this context means adapting my pace to Molly's. She is slower now. That is our reality. I'd better accept the fact that things take longer.

The next lesson I thought I'd learned involved adjusting my communication with Molly as she has lost more and more words. For the longest time, I thought my primary focus should be on decoding what she said. I started listening more carefully to every word, especially searching for substitutions she repeated. All children and babies became "little guys" early on. This term applied to children she didn't know, like those on the playground of the school we passed on our daily walks. It also referred to her nine-year-old grandson once she forgot his name.

This kind of interpreting was relatively easy. However, it became more challenging when Molly started using general terms like "thing" when she couldn't think of a word. Sometimes a word would occur to her completely out of context. The other day she pointed to our car and said, "Are we going to use the hat?"

That one came with a non-verbal clue so it wasn't very hard to figure out. More often I just couldn't understand what she was saying.

It was frustrating, too, because I could tell two important things: in her own head she was making sense, and she really did want to tell me something. Therefore, I worked extra hard at decoding as best I could.

What I missed in the effort to understand her side of the conversation was that she was also losing the ability to understand me. It took quite a while to realize that she didn't know what I was saying. After all, I have no aphasia. I was using the right words in the right contexts. She should still be able to understand me.

Not so. I started to notice that when I gave her simple instructions, "Get up. We're going now" or "Sit here," she didn't respond. Molly was not being stubborn: she just didn't remember the meaning of the words I was using. Repeating myself or employing different words wasn't going to work if she truly couldn't understand.

Finally I have learned to use many more non-verbal clues. Sometimes guiding her with touch. Sometimes modeling what it is I want her to do. Now, when we are trying to cross the street and a car is turning the corner and coming towards us, I just hug her until the vehicle passes. It always works.

TOUCH

Touch as Love

There is sight: the shine of a smile in her eyes.

There is hearing: the sound of our voices

Blending in an old song.

There are taste and smell:

We share treats and offer bits of food

To one another.

But for love the truest sense is touch:

Holding her hand is love.

Smoothing her hair is love.

Pressing my lips to hers is love.

Yes, as long as we can touch each other

We still have love.

Molly and I both loved the Winnie the Pooh stories from childhood and would sometimes read them to each other and laugh at all the silly parts. In one of the stories, Piglet, who is small and timid, takes Pooh's hand as they are walking home. Piglet says, "I want to be sure of you."

I can tell that Molly wants to be sure of me and I of her.

I hold Molly's hand much of the time when we are together, especially when we are out walking along the crazy busy avenue where she lives. I even hug her tightly when she wants to cross against the light and I see cars coming.

She holds onto my hand or my leg when we sit together and sing along to the musical performers on Mondays, Wednesdays, and Fridays. When it is chilly or windy, she often wears a hooded sweatshirt. When she puts the hood up, she pushes the hair back off her face. When I put the hood up for her, I get to smooth her hair. It feels soft and lovely.

When we take a rest in her room, we hold hands as we lie on her bed. I may think she has fallen asleep, but as soon as I move or get up, she springs to attention ready to go with me wherever.

When I am reading her a story, she often rubs my leg nearest her. Then I think, "Does she remember how we touched each other before? How comforting it could be, or how exciting?" Perhaps she does. That's a lovely thought.

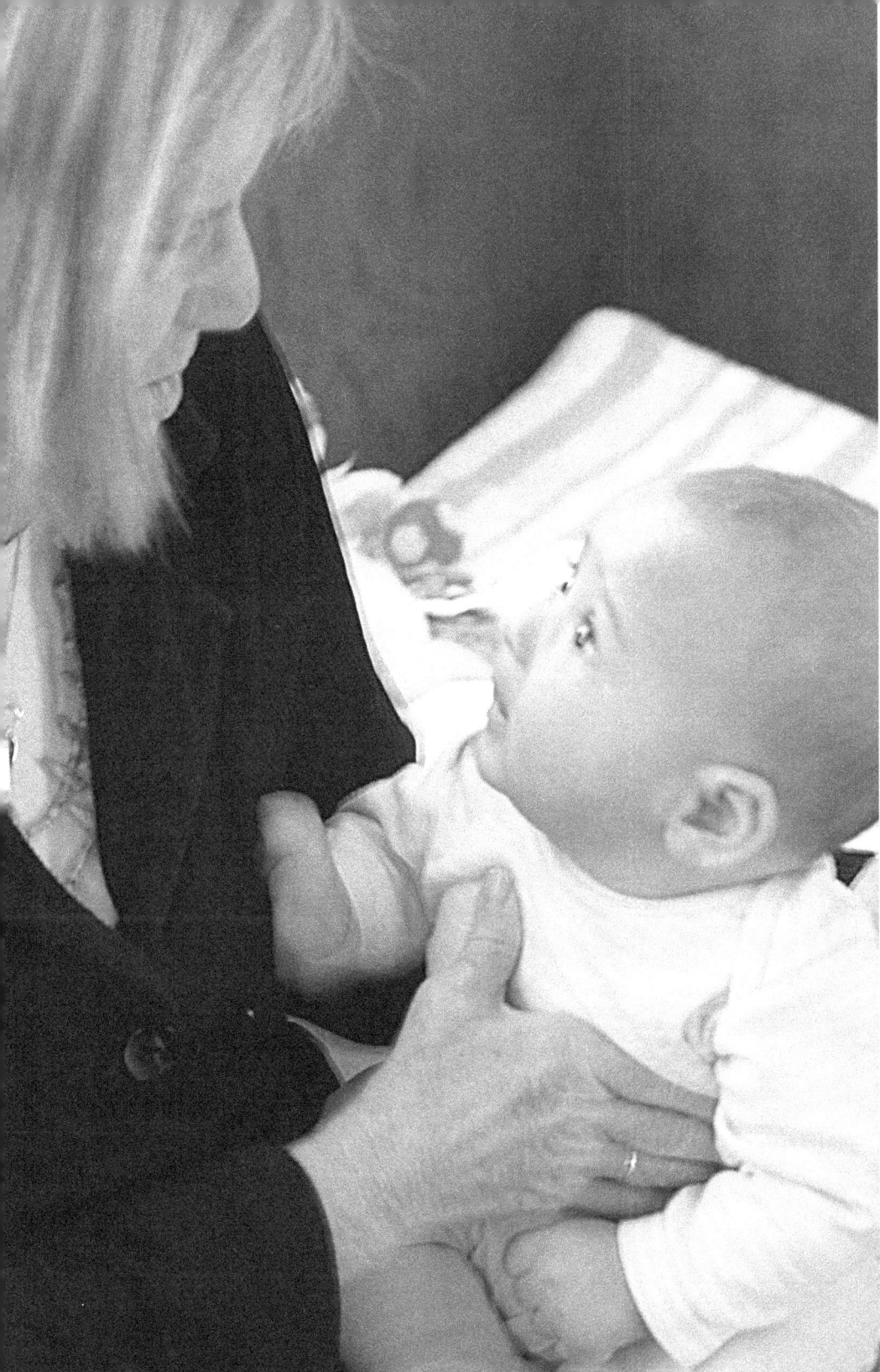

Molly with grandson Taj as a newborn.

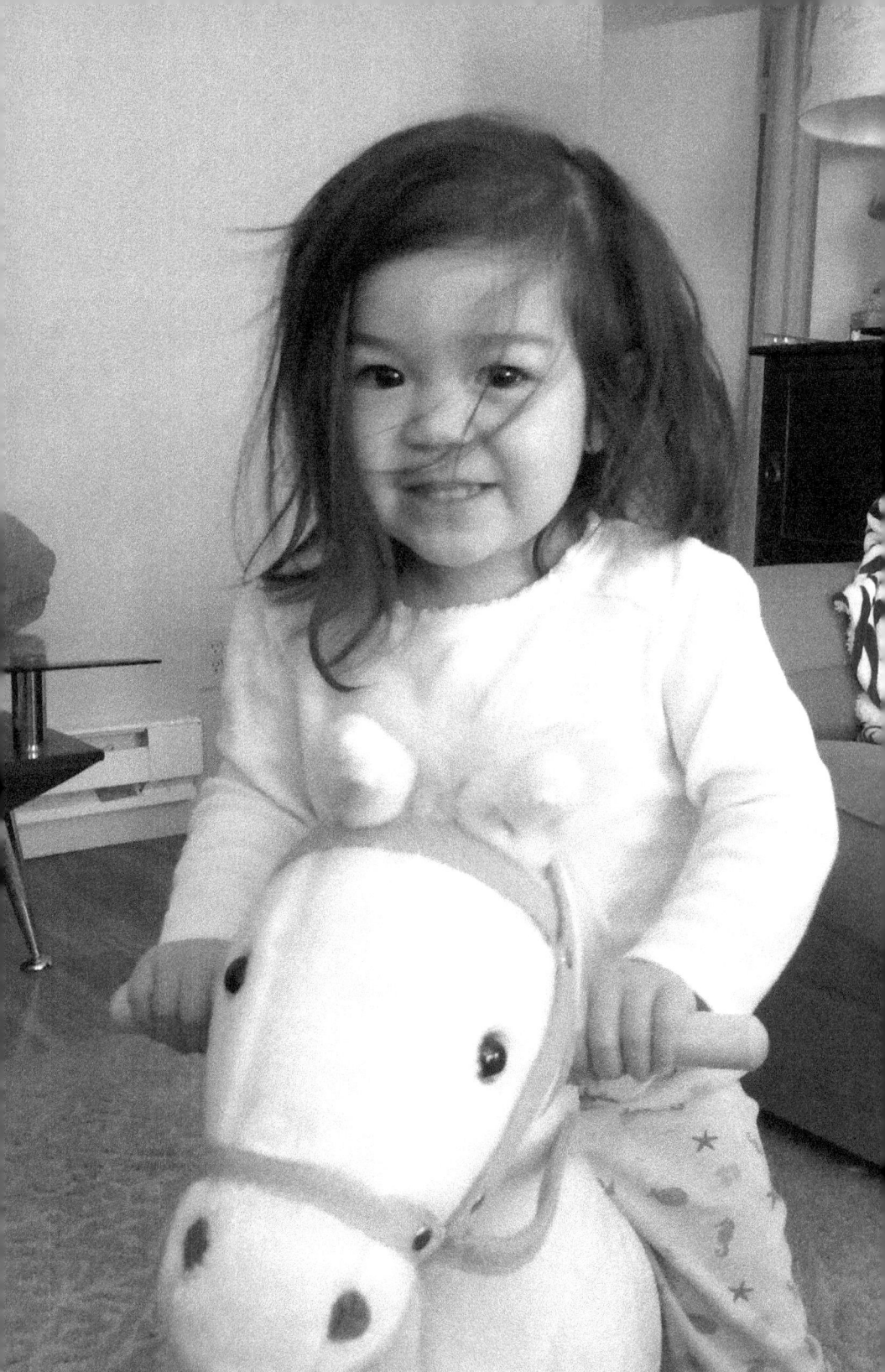

Molly granddaughter Sophia.

Part Two: New Normal

NOT PAPA

When I arrived today, Molly was sitting with a man in a U.S. Navy cap (we'll call him Mac). Mac is her special friend, and she spends a lot of time hanging out with him. After she greeted me, she went and sat down again, and I joined the two of them on the sofa. Molly said, "This is Papa," pointing to the man next to her.

Before I even thought, I blurted, "That is *not* Papa. This is Papa," pointing to myself. "That is Mac."

I know that she refers to all kinds of people, male and female, resident and staff, as "Papa." She's also called her son "Papa." It shouldn't matter at all, and yet at that moment it did matter.

She hasn't called me Willem for many months, so Papa is her name for me, and I want my name to be mine. It's one of the things I have left. When I no longer have a name, who or what will I be?

I grieve. It hurts already.

It reminds me of the time period when Molly and I were first married. We met as colleagues teaching at a college in New Jersey. Molly had already been there many years before I arrived, and she had tenure. We both had status as "Dr. O'Reilly" and "Dr. Oates."

I went through my tenure review the year we got together. I was denied tenure and given a one-year contract for the next year, after which I was terminated.

Molly, of course, stayed on, for another sixteen years after I left. During those years I experienced a loss of identity. Once I was let go, my status evaporated and I became an invisible person. (Perhaps some of Molly's colleagues thought my failure might be catching.)

I would go to meet Molly for lunch or to pick her up after class, and faculty members, my former colleagues, would pass me in the hallway without any recognition of my presence. To them, I no longer existed. At first I was mostly confused, and then I was hurt and angry. How was I different from the person who was their equal two semesters previously? I was still just as smart; I still had my Ph.D.; I still had ten years of experience as a college professor.

Now years later, I can look back and say with conviction, "Their snubbing me was their problem. Not mine."

Is this why Molly wanted to keep her diagnosis secret? Did she know somehow that a person with cognitive impairment would be less than a whole person? I think she did.

JEALOUSY DREAM

Early this morning, I had a dream. In it, Molly is with another man. He has placed an ad in the newspaper looking for a companion, and Molly has answered it. (People used to do such things: Molly and I often enjoyed reading the elaborate personal ads in *The New York Review of Books.*)

In my dream, Molly is in her house in a room with glass walls and a glass door. She and the man are sitting down at a table. Molly is wearing a pink coat, and it appears that she has nothing on underneath.

Her children come into the house and open the glass door. Her daughter says, "Mom, how can we know if you are . . . you know, busy?" Molly responds, "You'll see a lighted cigarette in the ashtray." She points to an ashtray on the table where smoke is rising from a burning cigarette.

The doorbell rings, and the daughter says, "Mom, you have to answer the door." Molly gets up and crosses the room. Her bare legs show beneath the pink coat.

At this point I awake from the dream.

I think I understand what prompted this dream. First, yesterday, the nurse at Molly's facility told me, "Molly is having a hard day. She was pressing her attentions on Mac, and he didn't want to be with her. So, he went to the other wing of the building. She became very aggressive and started hitting and kicking people." I couldn't help feeling a little pang of jealousy. Second, my friend Beth was asking me questions about Molly now. "Does she still recognize you? Does she know you're married? Does she understand that you have a new grandchild?" I replied, "I know she still recognizes me and calls me 'Papa.'" I wish I knew what she understands especially about family, but I don't and I never will. She can't tell me: either the memories are gone or she can't find the words.

Earlier this morning, I awoke and, half asleep, turned to where Molly would have been. Then I realized her side of the bed was empty.

It is March getting near to St. Patrick's Day, so I went to hear a concert by Danu, a band from Ireland. The lead singer did several songs in Irish. One song was about a young man who was sick in bed having lost his love, who was both beautiful and rich. The soloist translated the chorus for us, "It's far away you are," and she explained "That's how you say you miss someone in Gaelic."

I see Molly almost every day. I can hold her hand and hug her and give her a kiss. Yet there are times when I still feel "It's far away you are, Molly."

MOLLY AT 75

March 30, 2013

Molly turned 75 on Thursday. Many people commented that they "couldn't believe it" because she looks so young. She does, indeed, look much younger than almost all of the other residents. She still has about three inches of blond left from her last hair coloring. She has good skin and not too many wrinkles. Especially when she smiles, she could pass for someone ten years younger.

That's the outside. Inside her head, in her brain, she is older than she looks. Today, we went to a restaurant for lunch. She did quite well. However, she drank like there was no tomorrow: three large glasses of iced tea and three more of water. I took her to the bathroom twice.

When we got back, I asked the nurse, "Is there anything with her meds that makes her thirsty or gives her dry mouth?" "No," she said. "She always drinks everything we put in front of her, and when she finishes her drinks, she drinks someone else's. The issue is upstairs, I think, she doesn't know when to stop."

"Upstairs" I don't think Molly ever got it that it was *her* birthday. She sang along "Happy Birthday to Molly. Happy Birthday to you" and she added "And many more" each time. She smiled and enjoyed what was going on, but she did not register that everyone was looking at her when they sang.

One thing about a landmark birthday like 75 is that it leads to the inevitable question, "Will there be an 80th birthday?" I don't know, and that's a scary uncertainty.

Thinking about death in this society is often frightening. For some families, denial is their primary coping strategy. "Oh, Mom's not really that sick. She's just going through a hard time right now. She'll feel better next week or in a couple of weeks."

For some, panic over the coming loss starts even before the person dies. "What will we ever do without her? Dad will be devastated."

With certain illnesses, increasing pain may be the issue that comes up. "Doctor, she just can't stand it. You've got to do something. She needs more meds."

I've had all of these fears on certain days and, probably, a few more. Right now, watching Molly decline and seeing her fellow residents decline, I often have my doubts about an 80th.

So, what to do with the fears? The obvious answer is to enjoy the time she has left, every day of it, however many there may be. At Molly's facility there is live music at least three times per week. Yesterday's guest was especially good, and some of the tunes were quite danceable. I got Molly up, and we danced at the back of the room.

I noticed that sometimes she stumbled a little. Her balance is not what it used to be. Even a simple waltz has become an unfamiliar activity. Yet we didn't stop; we just held each other more tightly.

Describing the moment later, I said it was possible to experience both pain and joy at the same time. I was acutely aware of the symptoms of her decline. Yet it still felt very good to hold her in my arms.

DECLINE ALL AROUND

Molly sits at the table in the dining room where they put people who need assistance eating. Molly doesn't need much help, but she does spit out her food and she often spills things.

The other day there was a new person at the table (we'll call her Jenny). When I first came to the facility, Jenny was among the most vivacious of all the residents. She had a very expressive face and was filled with energy. She was always the first one up when there was the opportunity to dance. She grinned and winked and waved.

Now, she's having trouble swallowing. A nurse helps her eat lunch one spoonful at a time. Her face seems frozen and masklike. When I greet her, Jenny turns to look at me but her eye contact is off. It seems like the muscles in her face aren't behaving properly.

Later I thought, "This is really sad to see someone like Jenny, who was so lively, go into this phase of dementia." (I don't know her official diagnosis since it's confidential, of course.) Yet I also realized that my vibrational energy was still OK. I didn't automatically sink into the feeling of grief.

It's been over six months since Molly joined Jenny and the others. I've been a regular visitor long enough to see changes in many of the residents. Some, like Jenny, have passed into a different phase of the disease. They are slower, more fragile, less stable. It is sad, but it is not shocking.

Am I just getting used to seeing these people and their disabilities every day? Am I recognizing that there is more to Jenny and the others than their medical conditions? After six months, am I passing (at least for now) into the final stage of my own grieving: arriving finally at acceptance?

I think it's probably all of the above. I'm also aware of recognizing and accepting Molly's new normal. This is where she lives; she's not coming back "home" to where we lived together. The residents are her new companions, in many ways her new family. They are all like cousins who haven't seen each other for a long time but are still linked together.

When we go out for a walk, I sense that Molly recognizes her new home when we return. She used to be a bit leery about going in the front door of the facility. Not so any more. It's where we're going. It's getting back. It's home.

DRUGS AND BEHAVIOR

Today, when I went to pick up Molly, she was asleep in the exercise circle at 10:00 in the morning. I was surprised, and then I remembered that the nurses had told me they were upping her meds because of her aggressive behavior. "But I don't want her to be drugged out," I thought.

My position is definitely influenced by an old-fashioned notion of nursing homes, where all the patients are lined up in wheelchairs half-asleep and drooling. However, that's not the way things are done anymore, and if a facility tried to operate that way, the state regulators would be all over them.

That being said, the messages I've been getting from the nurses at Molly's facility are pretty clear and simple. Molly's aggression is causing problems for residents, staff, and visitors. The way to solve these problems is to give her higher doses of medications that lessen her aggression.

Today the on-duty nurse was talking about yet another increase. "We have to check with the doctor because we just increased her meds and we don't know if we can increase them again so soon."

If Molly is already falling asleep, what's she going to be like with more meds in her? I'd like to know what the alternatives are so I'm going to have to talk to her doctor myself, as well as get info from her doctor daughter and from friends who have some expertise.

I've generally been a minimalist on medications: less is more. In this case, however, I really don't know if that is the right perspective for Molly at this time in this place.

I did ask the nurse some questions to reassure myself about the immediate situation. "How long have you been here?" "Seven years." "So you've seen this before?" "Oh, yes." At least we are on the same page about Molly: this is a symptom of the disease. This is not the "real" Molly.

It's still important to me that other people see the good person I know Molly to be. Sometimes it seems like that's just my issue. Other times it seems significant: if the caregivers, in particular, see Molly as aggressive or even violent, they may not care for her as well.

When Molly first got to the unit, the Director told me that some of the staff were afraid of her. I thought the whole idea absurd, but I don't anymore. No one likes to be hit. No one likes to be spit upon. I have seen one staff member fumbling with her keys trying to open a door for me, because she was afraid of what Molly would do when I left.

Ah, yes, problems. Today one day after I found her asleep and started to doubt the future, things are much better. The caregiver from Shanghai gave her a bath and asked me to come and help. Molly doesn't like baths, and she HATES having her hair washed. Often she will go into a screaming fit. I can at least talk to her, tell her "You will be fine." "It is OK." "It will be over soon." "Almost done." Sometimes it helps; sometimes it doesn't.

Today she objected, but calmly, and looked at me with a roll-your-eyes look. She found the whole bathing thing unnecessary and annoying, but tolerable. Afterwards she smiled at the care partner and hugged her! She got a big, warm smile in return.

NEW BOYFRIEND

April 11, 2013

Among the fifty-two residents at Molly's facility, there is one longstanding couple (we'll call them Paul and Sandy). They always sit next to each other in the front row during the music events, often with Sandy's head on Paul's shoulder. They hug and kiss and dance together.

I have seen the staff struggle to separate them when Sandy's family came to take her out to lunch but she didn't want to go without Paul. I have been told that their families do not approve of their friendship and insisted on their rooms being in different wings. The practical implication is that they are often kept apart by locked doors, especially at meal times. Right now Paul is in Molly's wing, and he doesn't like the separation from Sandy.

After lunch, he was ready to see Sandy and went to the door and tried the handle several times. The care partner said, "The door will be open at 1:00, and she will be there." Paul looked puzzled. I could imagine him thinking, "What is 1:00? Why can't I see her now?"

The subject of Paul and Sandy came up this week when I met the wife of Molly's new special friend (we'll call him Tom and her Sophie). Previously Molly had spent a number of weeks clinging to Mac. She wound up getting quite possessive and would push people away who came between them. She even hit some people. Mac declared that Molly "was mean" and started staying away from her. So resourceful Molly latched onto Tom.

When I told Sophie about Paul and Sandy's being kept apart, she responded, "But that's just cruel." Sophie's position is that the residents, including Tom and Molly, should be allowed relationships that give them comfort and loving attention. Sophie related to me what happened when she first noticed Tom and Molly as a couple. "I was sitting with Tom when Molly came over and sat on the arm of Tom's chair. She patted him on the head. He doesn't let me do that anymore. Then she leaned over and kissed him on the top of his head and said, 'I love you.'" At the time Sophie was both upset and moved.

When we met, Sophie told me this story and said she was okay with what was going on between them. She said she hoped I would be, too. I said I was, in large part because I had had my little fling with jealousy over Mac, and also because Sophie was so clear about her feelings for Tom at this stage of his life. "He's not the man I married, but I will love him and try to make him happy 'til the day he dies."

Today at lunch I pulled up a chair where Tom and Molly were sitting. Molly was eating with her fingers. When she finished, Tom reached over with his bib and wiped off her hand. It was so sweet and caring that it was impossible not to see it as right.

A little bit later, when Molly got up to go with me, Tom rose to follow her. The care partner said very sternly several times, "Tom, sit down." Eventually he did. Ironically I felt for *him*. Why shouldn't Tom be allowed to follow Molly if he wanted to? He doesn't remember he's married to someone else, or what "married" means. Even if he were conscious of being married, his affection for Molly is both innocent and genuine. As is hers for him.

TOM AND SOPHIE

I keep in touch with Sophie, the wife of Molly's special friend, Tom. We try to time our visits so we are there at the same time. It's enough of a pattern that Tom has noticed. Yesterday when I arrived, he looked around and asked "Sophie?" wondering why she wasn't there when I was.

Today Sophie was there, and it was a beautiful day so we all wanted to be outside. Molly and I took our usual walk "around the block" (about seven blocks actually) with a stop at the coffee place. When I went to pay for the coffee, I realized I had left my wallet at home. Since we've been there so many times, the boy at the cash register just let me write an I.O.U.

When we got back, Sophie was ready to take Tom out. Tom had had a serious fall, so Sophie asked for a wheelchair. The four of us slowly circled the building getting a nice dose of fresh air. At the back of building where there is a driveway and no cutouts, Sophie and I worked together to lift Tom down off the curb and up on the other side.

Tom has more physical symptoms than Molly. He has a lot of trouble controlling his limbs. He still feeds himself, but it is a serious effort for him. I sit at the table between Tom and Molly repeating over and over to myself, "Don't do for him what he can do for himself." I mentioned to Sophie about watching Tom struggle while eating a piece of cake. She said, "Didn't they cut it up for him?" "No," I said, "and I didn't want to interfere." "Well, if it ever happens again, you have my permission to cut it up for him."

I've become attached to Tom. He is Molly's friend and my friend, too.

Tom has difficulty speaking as well, but when he does say something, it is quite clear. One day he looked at Molly and said, "How many children?" I explained the three older children and the three adopted ones, six total. He definitely understood.

I've only known him a few weeks, but I can sense the real Tom inside the ravaged body. He is funny and smart and strong willed.   He remembers some things very well. At one time he lived and worked in Chicago. Today in Colorado, it was spring-like with a breeze. Tom complained that it was cold. I commented, "I'll bet it's colder in Chicago." He laughed and said, "Yes, it is."

When he was in the wheelchair today, Tom looked smaller and more frail. I looked at him and thought, "Oh, my God, what if he has to move to skilled nursing, or what if he dies? Molly would miss him terribly."

"OK, Willem, no wild speculation about the future! Stay in the present. Enjoy the beautiful day. Be grateful that right now Tom and Sophie are in Molly's life and yours."

I came back to reality. It was still a very beautiful spring day; I was truly grateful.

MEN'S GROUP

In Boulder we have every kind of group imaginable: there is a cosmology group that studies the physics of the Universe; there is a Women of the West book club that focuses on female authors; there is a world politics group that covers current events every Tuesday. These are just a few examples of those at the public library.

So, it's no surprise that there are multiple men's discussion groups. Two of these groups are part of a larger movement we'll call HIStory. HIStory runs men's weekend retreats and weekly groups. After completing my first piece of writing "An Open Letter to Men Who Are Caregivers," I thought about participating in HIStory.

I e-mailed my piece to the group leader, and he wrote back enthusiastically inviting me to speak at the next meeting. When I got there, I met everyone and we all checked in.

When my turn came to speak, I read my piece, "I am a caregiver, and I am a man. . . ." Everyone was impressed and gave positive feedback. It turned out that of the nine men there, three of us were, or had recently been, primary caregivers for our wives.

Then I talked about my immediate fears. Just the day before I had found out that Molly's special friend Tom had gone on hospice. I knew that meant he had less than six months to live. Tom was going to die and soon. And, if Tom was going to die, then Molly was going to die.

I let my emotions show and cried several times. I was used to sharing my feelings in my Twelve Step meetings and felt it would be equally safe with this group.

However, after I finished the guy sitting directly across from me said, "I liked the way you let your mask down. But then I saw it go up again."

I replied, "Well, I am new here and I don't know any of you. I was as open as I could be, and then I needed to stop. Since I'm so new to this group, I'm sure you can cut me some slack."

The therapist who runs the group spoke up. "I don't care for that remark. These men are offering you love, and when you make a joke you are disrespecting them."

I was speechless for a few moments, but not for long. "I feel that you have just shamed me." The therapist sputtered, "Is there anything I can do for you right now?"

I closed my eyes. When I opened them and opened my mouth, the right answer poured out. "Yes, you could do something to fix me, and it might even work—temporarily—but it wouldn't be right. I am responsible for my own feelings. If I'm feeling ashamed, them it's my job to tell myself that I am OK."

I did just that, and it felt *wonderful*.

ST. MICHAEL

I dream, and in the dream I am in a large building like a warehouse. There are objects lying on the floor. They are shaped like torpedoes—cylindrical on one end and flat like an oar at the other end.

There are other people there. Our task is to find two of the objects that match.

I must have done so, for I next see myself in a church pew with two of the objects standing up behind me. The "sculpture" is very tall–nine or ten feet high—and the flat parts resemble angels' wings.

I cannot see anything beyond the object and myself.

Then a young woman with yellow curly hair and a halo of light around her head emerges. Her face is beautiful and glowing.

She speaks, "St. Michael is the ultimate proof of the existence of God. If he exists, then God exists."

I awaken and think, "What's this about St. Michael? What does this warrior archangel who fought Satan have to do with me?"

I Google St. Michael, and I find out that in the early Christian church St. Michael was the Patron of Sickness. People prayed to him to be healed of illnesses.

Now I know why I had the dream about this Archangel.

WALKING OUT WITH MOLLY

In the Buddhist tradition one meditates on the five remembrances, which include: "I am of the nature to age. I am of the nature to get sick. I am of the nature to die."

Where I live in Boulder, Colorado, there are many, many people on the jogging trails and at the gyms and out on their bikes who are trying their best to believe the opposite.

Molly and I followed a pretty healthy lifestyle though we were neither as dedicated nor as obsessive as some of our friends and neighbors. Early on when we still lived in New Jersey, we got in the habit of taking long walks along the canal path that had been reborn as a hiking and biking trail. When we moved to Colorado twelve years ago we took advantage of the opportunity to hike in some of the most glorious places in the country.

Molly got very fit.

When Molly was in her wandering phase we found out how fit. One day she disappeared, and we called the police to help us find her. The Sheriff's Department had in fact attached a tracking device to her ankle so we thought it would be easy to find her. The device never did work properly, however, and it was good luck that a police car happened to see her on the side of the road about four miles from our house.

I have no idea where Molly thought she was going, but she really moved once she got started.

Today I was reading some materials on the later stages of Alzheimer's. One of the key factors is reaching the point where one can't walk. You are stuck in bed or perhaps a chair, and the end is near.

When Molly first got to the facility, her level of activity was of concern to the staff. "She goes so fast we can't keep up with her," one would say. "The way she moves up and down the hall, she could knock over one of the elder residents."

When I visit, I make a point of walking with her every time. Unless it's snowing or under 30 degrees. What I have noticed is that she walks just fine but now has a little trouble with stairs. I asked the personal trainer who has many clients at the facility about that. "Oh, yes," she said, "if you stop doing something you lose the muscle memory of how to do it."

Another kind of "memory" that Molly is losing.

This is, indeed, a terrible disease.

I see the inevitable decline in the other residents. Some have gone from walking to shuffling in the last few months. It is very easy for me to go down the rabbit hole of the future and see Molly that way.

But, no. In the present, Molly is still healthy. Right now she walks with a firm stride.

And I am grateful for every step.

MOLLY DOESN'T KNOW ME

April 25, 2013

It was hard with Molly today. I was gone for a week visiting my family in Chicago on the occasion of my Mother's 89th birthday.

When I came in Molly was sitting with Mac watching TV, not Tom but Mac again. She didn't get up to greet me, so I went to the sofa and sat next to her.

WILLEM: Let's go hear the music. (I point towards the Town Square room where musicians perform.)
MOLLY: No, I can't do that. (She has a determined look in her eyes. Her body is rigid.)
WILLEM: You can come with me.
MOLLY: No.
WILLEM: Do you want to go for a walk? (Pause.) Or, do you want to stay here?
MOLLY: Stay here.
WILLEM: You could come with me.
MOLLY: No, I can't do that.

"Oh my God," I think. "She has forgotten who I am in the week I was gone." I start to tear up but hold back. I never cry in front of Molly.

I think, "If she just sees the front door, she'll want to go out. She always does."

WILLEM: Mac, would you come with us? (I want Molly to go to the front door.)
MAC: This is your Dad. (Mac gets up, but Molly stays seated. Then she rises. She clings to Mac.) This is your . . . husband. (He pushes Molly away forcefully.) (Angrily.) I will kill you.

(Molly stands silent and stunned. Finally she turns to follow me. We leave the room and head for the exit door. Mac is standing watching us go.)

When we get outside, Molly softens and lets me take her hand. I have a knot in my stomach. I start to sing "When you wore a tulip . . ." She joins in, and I begin to calm down. Three times through "Tulip" and once through "Bicycle Built for Two" and we are back to *normal*—whatever the heck that is.

My thoughts are racing: "That was really scary. Could she possibly have been punishing me for being gone so long? This is what it will be like when she doesn't recognize me. I don't like it at all. When will it happen? Will it be soon?"

After I have been with her for about three hours, Molly is clinging to *me*. When I try to leave, she follows me and I can hear her at the door jiggling the handle and knocking. I stop to use the restroom. When I come out, there is Molly with a care partner right behind her. "We found her in the kitchen."

Molly somehow got through a locked door to find me. Nora, her daughter, would be proud of her spunk.

EASY FOR ME

I am on the phone with my friend Beth. "Today is the first day Molly ignored me completely. She was with Mac, and she didn't want to do anything with me." Beth replied, "She's certainly making it easy for you, isn't she?"

Beth was referring to a new emotional attachment in my life. We'll call her Patricia. I met her through my sister. She is also a writer, and we exchanged pieces and started to talk. She lives in the Chicago area where my Mother and ten of my siblings are.

While I was in Chicago I went on a "date" with Patricia. We went to see a play adapted from a book entitled *Still Alice*. *Still Alice* follows the decline of a woman who develops early onset Alzheimer's at age fifty. Like Molly, Alice is a university professor, and it is particularly tragic for her husband and children to see a brilliant mind disintegrate. I related completely.

The play was very well done; the acting was superb. In particular, the woman who played Alice disappeared so fully into her character that we, in the audience, saw only Alice. We were watching the real Alice: this is how Alice walks and talks and behaves.

I cried, of course, responding to the many parallels in the story between Alice and Molly. At one point near the very end of the play, Alice's husband John says to her, "You were the smartest woman I ever knew."

I have often said the exact same words about Molly, and I wept at the loss of such talent and sparkling intelligence.

Patricia and I saw each other two more times during my visit to Chicago. We continued to correspond and talk on the phone and Skype. Patricia saw me as her friend's brother and a fellow writer, but at one point she said, "I didn't know I was going to like you so much." I was getting closer to her every day, every week.

Meanwhile, Molly was making it "easy" for me. First she had attached herself to Mac. Then when Mac backed away, she found Tom. Whatever is going on in what is left of Molly's mind, she needs male companionship. When I am not around, she finds another man to be with. She is very affectionate with her special friends.

Gradually I have come to accept this new normal. Sometimes Molly responds to me in the old way: she is happy to see me and spend time with me. We go for a walk, hold hands and sing together. She tells me she loves me.

Other times she seems not to recognize me. Rather she wants to be with Mac or Tom when I visit. When I ask her to go for a walk, she says, "I can't do that."

So Molly and I are in a real sense "separated." We no longer live together. We have not had sex for more than a year and a half. She spends much of her time with other men.

But does that really make me free to commit emotionally to someone new? Maybe yes, maybe no. Most days I feel OK with building a relationship with Patricia. Other days I feel GUILTY as hell.

Patricia says "It's complicated." How right she is.

MOLLY AND MAC, CAROL AND I

I've been back from my trip to Chicago for four days, and Molly is different each time I visit. The first time she seemed not to know me.

Today Molly ignored me at first. She was with Mac when I arrived, and her attention was on him. I asked her if she wanted to go for a walk. She said, "Can he come, too?" I started to say "No" since I'm not permitted to take anyone but Molly out of the facility. Then I noticed that one of the care partners was taking a group out for a walk around the building.

I led Molly and Mac out to join this group. They were holding hands and walking in front of me. The care partner (we'll call him Benjamin) was at the back of the group with two women who move more slowly. He took the hand of the last woman in the group and asked me to hold onto the other woman (we'll call her Carol).

Carol is a sweet little lady with a lovely smile. I know her a little bit because when I first started visiting she mistook me for her son. "Are you John?" she would ask when I arrived. "No, but I do look a lot like him." That would satisfy her, and she would smile at me warmly. I liked being on the end of that smile and made a point of greeting her even when she stopped thinking I was her son.

I took Carol's hand and fell in behind Molly and Mac. I had a little twinge of jealousy seeing Molly so content walking hand-in-hand with Mac. However, it passed because Carol was so grateful to have my strong presence with her. At one point she stumbled a bit. I don't think she would have fallen, but she thanked me for holding her up. I smiled.

We circled the building once, and circled it again. It was a beautiful spring day, the first one where the temperature hit 70 degrees. The trees were beginning to go from bud to leaf, and the forsythia bushes were showing the first bits of yellow. No one wanted to go back inside.

When we did go back inside, there was still about half an hour to go before everyone took their places for dinner, so we sat and watched a video on life in the ocean around the Bahamas. I was sitting with Carol. Molly was a few seats over with Mac. At one point Molly leaned forward to look and see where I was so she did know that I was there.

Once we got into the dining room, routine took over and Molly acknowledged my presence. I sat next to her and cut her food into smaller bites. She shared her dessert cookie with me. She checked my coffee cup to see if I was finished the way she always does.

Later we saw Tom, Molly's other special friend, with Deirdre, his agency caregiver. Deirdre asked me to help her take Tom to the bathroom. I knew what to do, but, even though he has lost weight, Tom felt quite heavy when we were lifting him in and out of his wheelchair.

Deirdre and I laughed at how futile some of our efforts were. Tom ignored the handicapped bar and instead held onto his pants with an iron grip. Our obvious powerlessness over his strong will just made us laugh more.

I left the facility thinking, "It's clear why I was here today. I needed to be here to help Carol and Tom and Deirdre." It felt very satisfying. A good day.

GOODYE TO TOM AND SOPHIE

April 15, 2013

Today, Tom was moved to a skilled nursing facility at 2:00 p.m.

Up until about three weeks ago Tom was healthy enough to stay in the memory-care unit with hospice visiting him there. Then he took a sudden turn for the worse. All of a sudden he couldn't maintain his balance. He had several bad falls. The last one resulted in bruises all over his body, including his face.

Sophie realized that Tom was now in the final phase of the disease and had decided Tom needed the extra attention he'd get in skilled nursing.

When I arrived on Tom's moving day, he was in his usual seat at the table where he and Molly usually eat lunch. However, Molly wasn't in her accustomed chair.

Tom had a caregiver feeding him the raw vegetables he likes. And Sophie arrived with her takeout lunch.

Sophie surveyed the scene and asked about Molly. "Oh, she's over there watching TV with Mac," I responded. Sophie rolled her eyes, "It's a new adventure every day. Isn't it?"

It sure is.

A little while later, Molly and I were in the lobby of the facility where they have space for activities, including the day's musical guest.

Tom came by in his wheelchair, and I shook his hand and said I would visit him. I never cry in front of Molly, but I did this time.

As Tom's wheelchair rolled through the front door for the last time, Molly got up to follow him. I told her a white lie, "Don't worry. They're only going out for a ride."

WISHING MOLLY DEAD

My psychiatrist has been telling me to "get on with my life" for years now. I had told her I was interested in a woman from my book club, and she encouraged me to build that relationship since Molly could no longer meet my needs.

That relationship only got so far, but the last time I saw my Doctor, I told her that I had met someone with whom I could see a long-term relationship and even marriage after Molly is gone. She was happy for me.

All of this took on a new perspective and intensity this week when Sophie transferred Tom to skilled nursing and talked about the end stage of his life. One of the things she said (and she had said it before) was, "Tom now is not the man I married twenty-one years ago. That person is gone."

That made me think hard about Molly. She is certainly not the person I married twenty-nine years ago.

I still think there is something left of the old Molly. But is that true? Or only an illusion on my part?

When I came back last week from my trip to Chicago, she didn't seem to recognize me at first. What is still left inside? Is the Molly I see today merely what I remember about her and project onto her?

She remembers old songs. I think mostly ones she learned with her father when she was young. She has no trouble with the words to "A Bicycle Built for Two." She enjoys the Winnie-the-Pooh stories we used to read to our children and sometimes to each other. She sings along with the traditional hymns at the religious services at the facility.

There are a few verbal things that she still remembers. One of them is taken from Oscar Wilde's play *The Importance of Being Earnest*, our favorite. In it, the leading character has a calling card that gives his address as "B-4, The Albany" (Hotel). We used to riff on that by saying "B-*fun*, the Albany." Now if I say something will "B-fun," Molly will still fill in "the Albany."

That's nice and makes me smile, but it's not much by way of conversation.

Bottom line then: is Molly essentially just as missing to me as Tom is to Sophie?

And if so, is it OK to "get on with my life?"

Even deeper and more deeply scary is the possibility that there is a part of me that wishes Molly dead so I can have a new life? Whoa. That is certainly someplace I don't want to go. I couldn't possibly still be a good person if that were true.

At the Conference on World Affairs at C.U. Boulder, there was a panel entitled "What Makes a BFF, What Makes a Soulmate." I went to the mike in the Q & A and asked "What if your soulmate is gone? My wife has Alzheimer's, and she is no longer with me." One of the experts on the panel responded, "Sometimes in a case like this, I put aside my role as a therapist and adopt a clerical position. I give you absolution. Go out and find love in your life."

Is that really OK? If I do that, I'll have to give up my story about being a good person because I'm still taking such good care of Molly. Letting go of that story will not be easy.

SAINTHOOD

Todd, one of the baristas at the coffee place where Molly and I go every day, asks me about Molly. "How much cognitive functioning does she still have?" I explain about Molly's aphasia and how she still talks but makes no sense most of the time. About how she hasn't been able to read and write for a long time. About how she most often doesn't understand what I say and just answers "Yes" to everything.

After I finish, he says, "You are a saint."

I squirm inside and mumble a thank you.   I don't feel like a saint, like St. Francis or Mother Theresa, people who have done truly extraordinary things, and, in the eyes of the Church, people who performed miracles that defy scientific explanations.

I am, I think most of the time, a relatively ordinary, loving husband whose wife is sick. I have taken care of her and continue to do what I can to make her day-to-day life a little happier.

I see many caregivers around me just as dedicated and loyal, just as loving, just as noble. It's part of the deal with dementia. We do a lot for the person with the disease because he or she needs a lot of help and we are the ones available to help.

I'm not at all comfortable with the saint label. But on the other hand I do visit Molly every day when I am not traveling. With a little effort, I can estimate the number of visits. Day 223 minus the first seventeen days (when I wasn't allowed to see her) and later when I went to see my new granddaughter and when I went to Chicago for my Mother's birthday, etc. There have been about fifty days I've missed. Total visits then approximately 173.

That's a pretty big number. Does it qualify me for sainthood? Not really. But it does qualify me as a *good person*.

Ah, now we're getting to the heart of the matter. A really good person keeps his loved one at home until the very end. I had the Director of a home care agency tell me this was possible before I placed Molly in the unit. That's what I would have done if I were a saint.

But, at least, I can still be a good person and visit every day.

Unfortunately, there is a part of me that still has something to prove, still needs to earn good person points. Yet another part of me knows full well that this is not healthy thinking and behavior.

This morning while I was meditating, this issue came up and I thought, "Well, I'm not perfect." Almost immediately, another thought arose, "Yes, you are." That second thought arises out of my work with A Course in Miracles. "You are as God created you." I was created perfect in God's eyes, and I am always so.

I don't have to earn any more points. I'm already more than OK. I may, in fact, be a saint.

UNCONDITIONAL LOVE

I spent time this weekend with my son Reynor, my daughter-in-law Adrienne, and my three-year-old grandson Taj. I wrote to my friend Beth about what a wonderful time I was having and how much I love Taj. She wrote back and noted that such love was "unconditional."

That made me think about the usual description of unconditional love. It's what a mother feels for her child. No matter what the child does—good, bad, or indifferent—the mother always loves the child. Very often in conversation the emphasis is on the bad: My son is using drugs, but I still love him. My daughter flunked out of school, but I still love her.

Molly and I certainly practiced this version with our adopted children. We have loved our adopted son, D.J., in particular, through over twenty years of rehabs and hospitals and courts and jails.

As for Taj, I find myself applying the no-matter-what principle to him, too. Sure he has tantrums. Sure he's sometimes aggressive. Sure he's stubborn . . . But I love him anyway. After all, isn't that what unconditional love means?

I said so in a reply to Beth. She responded with "By unconditional, I also mean love that is eternal for everyone that we can always dip into. In a way, it's like we live in two worlds." She was coming at the definition from an entirely different place, from a spiritual perspective.

It reminded me of some of the religious teachings we got as children. One had to do with Mary, the Mother of Jesus. We were all praying to her, and she was supposed to love all of us. But how was it possible to love so many people all over the world?

The standard answer was that Mary was like a giant pitcher of love. Whenever she poured out some for one of us, the pitcher (magically) filled up again. Mary's pitcher of love was always full.

Beth was suggesting that each of us has the same capacity for love that we as children imagined for Mary. We can all access love directly from the source, God or Spirit or Creator or Light.

There's never a shortage. We never have to worry about giving or receiving enough love.

I have to admit I've never thought of love this way. When I was growing up there was a new baby every year until we hit fourteen children. There was never enough of anything, especially mother love.

This came up when I was doing my Al-Anon Fifth Step. The Fifth Step states "We admitted to God, ourselves and another human being the exact nature of our wrongs."

In my Fifth Step process, I followed a method that helps us identify beliefs we have about ourselves that are not true.

This method divides the false self beliefs into five categories, including Addiction/Spirituality. This one suggests that we use our addiction of choice—alcohol or drugs or food or sex or work—as a means to fill up a hole in our souls.

I think we also use our addiction of choice to fill a parallel hole in our hearts.

We who felt such holes didn't believe in the unconditional love to which Beth referred. Rather we felt that there was never enough, that we were not getting what we needed.

At the end of the Fifth Step process on this issue, I wrote the false statement "I am outside the circle of love." Then below it I wrote "THIS IS A LIE."

I am, in fact, always connected to unconditional love. I have felt it with Molly. I am beginning to feel it for myself. My life is so much richer now that I share unconditional love with Taj.

CARE CONFERENCE

May 10, 2013

After Molly has been a patient in the memory-care unit for eight months, her six-month care conference was finally scheduled.

I followed advice and wrote down the points I wanted to cover, but there was really only one big issue. It is a very big one: Molly is more aggressive, sometimes violent, and the staff—in concert with the doctor—want to solve this problem with medications that calm her down.

I want to minimize her meds so she is not sleeping too much. I will have to negotiate a compromise. I use the line "I don't want her to be a zombie" very often in these negotiations.

Vis a vis compromise, the meeting went pretty well. We all agreed that Molly's hitting other residents was over the line. The increased dosage of the antipsychotic Seroquel seemed to be having a positive effect. Of course, Tom's absence is also a major factor. Molly can no longer cause him to fall because she walks too fast.

I am often in the position of not knowing what has been happening. This frustrates me greatly. "Oh, we couldn't tell you about that because of HIPPA (the federal privacy rules)." At one point, the Director actually turned to me and said, "You have to be realistic." How can I be expected to be realistic about Molly's behavior when no one will tell me what she did?

Another completely absurd encounter occurred with one of the nurses who described Molly's spitting out her morning meds. "She was transitioning from breakfast to the exercise circle, and the care partner gave her the meds in a spoon. Molly always takes them in her hand." The nurse demonstrated how Molly normally pops the meds into her mouth. "But they [the staff] will learn." "If she keeps spitting out her meds, they'd better learn," I responded.

But, wait a minute. The nurses supervise the care partners. Why would the nurse let the care partner learn about Molly by trial and error when she, the nurse, already knows the right way to handle Molly??

Sometimes I really don't understand what the heck is going on.

I was dissatisfied enough to call the Director the next day and talk things over on the phone. She explained that the "realistic" comment referred to the staff growing accustomed to Molly's aggressive behavior. "They get numb to it, so they don't report it."

Yes, Molly is more aggressive: she needs to take more meds. I get it. We have reached yet another new normal.

Yes I, Willem, will continue to advocate as hard as I can for the best quality of life Molly can have in her current condition.

The bottom line is that the staff and I have agreed to disagree. I suppose that counts as a "realistic" compromise.

MOTHER'S DAY

May 12, 2013

Today is Mother's Day. I picked up Molly from the facility and took her to her son Chris's house for waffles. We had planned this over the phone, and he asked if she would be OK. I told him she'd be fine with driving in the car, but she would eat with her hands. "That's normal around here," he said.

The only accommodation I had to make was to cut the waffles into quarters. Molly picked them up, ate them, and enjoyed herself.

Then we went for a walk across the park and down a trail adjacent to Chris's subdivision. Molly was fine for about twenty minutes going and coming back. Then suddenly she lost it. She started staggering and gasping for breath, and I had to support her to keep her from falling.

I kept pointing to the house and our car parked in front. "There, you see. We're almost there." I repeated this several times before I realized that her head was sagging, her eyes downward, and there was no way she could look ahead to see our goal.

We made it back, and I installed her on the sofa and got her water. She relaxed and seemed better almost immediately although she did spill the water.

After the spill I took her to the bathroom and changed her wet Depends. Was it just time for a change after breakfast, or had she wet herself in panic as we crossed the park? No way to know.

What was clear was that we were experiencing yet another symptom of decline. This summer there will probably be shorter and shorter walks as she inevitably loses more mobility. I hate this terrible disease.

However, the day got much better when we returned to the facility for the Mother's Day tea. Many family members (children and grandchildren and great grandchildren, even a set of three-month-old twins) visited. The food was delicious. Everyone was smiling and talking and taking pictures.

Molly and I sat with B.J. and two of her three daughters, Sally and Mary. Mary had a new iPad, and I used it to take a great picture of the three of them. Later, when things got too noisy, we went out into one of the patio gardens. It was a perfect spring day outside with the sky a brilliant Colorado blue.

I had made up my mind to sing "Any Man Who Loves His Mother" at some point. It's a rat pack song from a Frank Sinatra movie called "Robin and the Seven Hoods." My Mother loved it and always insisted on hearing it any time my four brothers and I were together. I warmed up with "When You Wore a Tulip," since this is one of B.J.'s favorites, and one of Molly's favorites, too. She and B.J. both sang along.

Then I did the "Mother" number. My Mother, a thousand miles away, is now eighty-nine years old. B.J. is eighty-eight. Coincidence? Not really.

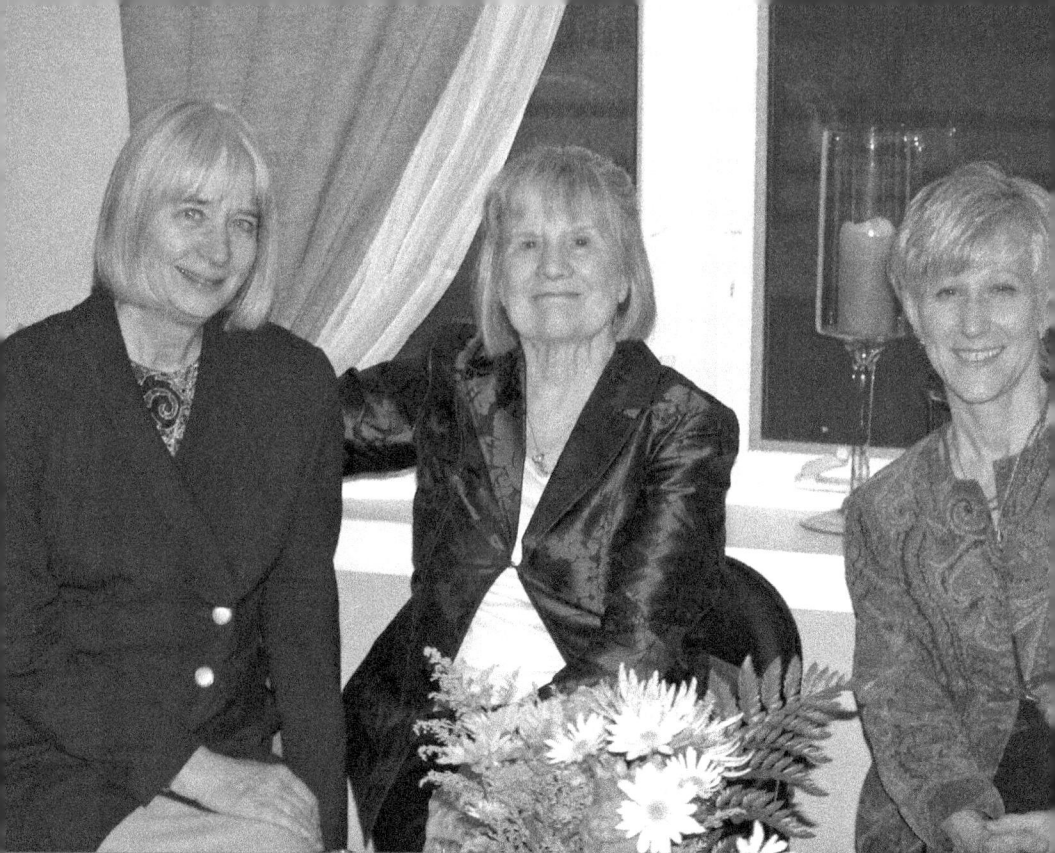

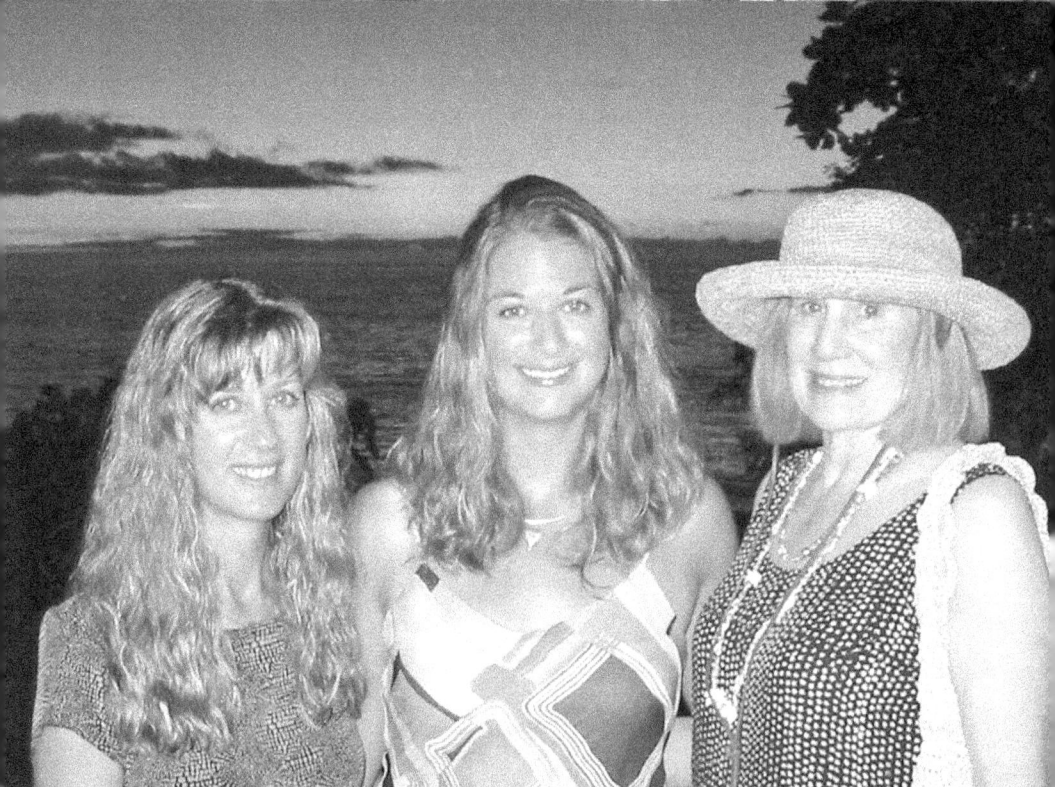

Molly with her professor colleagues Dr. Judith Johnson and Dr. Roberta Sethi at 25th anniversary party in 2009.
Molly with daughter-in-law Adrienne and Adrienne's mother Mona Bellantonio in Hawaii 2007.

ANOTHER NEW NORMAL

Most days when I go to visit Molly now, I don't know how she will react. Some days she greets me with a big smile and is eager to be with me. We go for a walk, sing songs, stop for coffee and a treat: pumpkin bread with chocolate chunks is her favorite.

Other times she's sitting with Mac and hardly notices my arrival. When I ask her if she'd like to go for a walk, she says, "I can't do that" and folds her arms across her chest.

Any jealousy on my part is a waste of energy. I know she doesn't know what's going on. I know she's not snubbing me on purpose. Her attention is just on Mac right then or on a TV show they are watching together.

What is my role then? I have evolved into an unofficial volunteer. The staff all know me very well, and so do the residents. Although I don't know all fifty residents' names, I'm working on learning them.

I have ridden on the twelve-person bus and helped with fastening seatbelts. I have served sundaes as part of a homemade ice cream project, for which I also turned the crank. I have walked around the building holding Carol's hand. I have danced with another resident when Molly wasn't interested.

I have played a lot of Bingo since Bingo is a regular weekly activity. The residents like it because the prizes are small chocolate candies. Some of them can follow the game just fine on their own, but many, including Molly, can't recognize the numbers on the card. If Molly wants to play, I sit next to her and keep my own card. Then I let her choose a chocolate when I get Bingo.

Yesterday was the first time I played without Molly. When I arrived, she was watching "Bonanza" reruns with Mac and didn't want to go for a walk.

As I walked away from Molly and Mac, I saw Paul and Peggy in the corridor trying different door handles. They were clearly looking for privacy, but neither one had a key to any of the rooms. So I did something naughty: I opened the door to Molly's room for them and let them in. Paul thanked me. What they did in Molly's room behind closed doors is their business. I had a mischievous grin on my face.

I went to the dining room where the Bingo game was already in progress. I found an open place at a table for four next to Carol. I figured she'd need help, and I was right. I kept one card myself and helped the others. When I won, I would donate my chocolate to someone who hadn't won yet. It was fun. When the leader of the activity was called away briefly, I called out the numbers as well.

Later, I helped one of the caregivers give Molly a bath. Many of the caregivers believe, and I think it's true, that I have a calming influence on Molly. I talk to her and tell her, "Almost done" and so on. Even with me there, Molly still did some hitting and screaming, but nothing too extreme.

For now (this month?) my "volunteering" is part of my new normal. I don't know how Molly will behave on any given day, but I'm not prepared to stop visiting. I participate in the activities of the day. I hang out with the residents I know and like.

It's a win-win for the residents and for me.

TOM DIED

May 20, 2013

Tom died last night.

I got the news in an email from Sophie.

I am crying as I write this, which sometimes happens. I find that when I am emotional I can still write if I say the words out loud while I type.

Despite the tears I was able to write back to Sophie with a special memory of Tom and Molly, a memory of the time when Tom wiped off Molly's hands with his bib after she had been eating with her fingers. It was a sweet moment—soft, gentle, loving.

I am aware of the five stages of grief so definitively described by Elisabeth Kübler-Ross in her book *On Death and Dying*. I can certainly relate to the first stage, denial. A big part of me says, "This is impossible. I just saw Tom a couple of weeks ago. I know he was on hospice, but he was supposed to be with us for six more months, not six weeks."

I also feel guilty since I never got to visit him at the skilled nursing facility.

When Sophie told me she had put Tom on hospice (I remember the day Monday and the date April 15), the emotion that gripped me was fear. "If Tom is really going to die and soon, then Molly is going to die and sooner than I think."

I was able to face that fear in part by writing about it, in part, by recognizing it and sharing it in my Twelve Step meeting.

Now I feel like jumping to Kübler-Ross's fifth stage, acceptance. Tom was in pain. His quality of life had declined drastically. He needed assistance with everything. He was sick and tired. It was his time to pass on. He didn't need to suffer any more. Sophie understood and let go of him. I believe he understood deeply that she accepted his going.

I hope to have the same grace and love Sophie had when my time comes with Molly. Sophie is my hero and my role model for loving at the end of life.

This very special case brings up the issue of death among Molly's new "family." These are the people she lives with now. She is fond of them. They are fond of her. I am fond of them. They are part of my life, too.

Who will be the next to die? What kind of hole will that leave? I do not like these thoughts. Maybe, they are unique to today and the shock of hearing about Tom. I sure hope so.

I know I need to feel this sadness: there is no avoiding it; running away does not help. Yet, right now, I want to run as fast and as far as I can.

IT HAPPENED TODAY

May 30, 2013

People ask all the time, "Does she still recognize you?" "Oh, yes," I say. "She still knows that I am a friend, and she is happy to see me. What she knows about 'married' or 'husband' I can't say."

That was until yesterday; now I'm not so sure. When I arrived at the facility a sing-a-long was already in progess.

With Tom gone, Molly is back to hanging out with Mac. Molly was sitting with Mac, so I sat in the row in front of them and joined the singing. I thought to myself, "She'll want to go for a walk after the songs."

When we got to "When You Wore a Tulip," one of our three sing-every-day songs, I turned around and said, "You know this one" and tried to get her to sing with me. She gave me a half smile.

After the sing-a-long, they served snacks, and I moved to a seat next to her. I asked her if she wanted to go for a walk. "No, I can't do that." I thought, "I'll just wait."

After the yogurt cups, I tried to entice her into going for a walk. I tried everything that had always worked before. I pointed to the front door and said, "Do you want to go there?" I used our code phrase "out and about." I started to sing "Bicycle Built for Two." Nothing worked.

Molly was standing with Mac; her back was to me; and there was a shadow on her overalls. I thought she might be wet, and I touched her to check. She said, "No, no, no," to my touching her. A few moments later, she left the room holding onto Mac. I got in the car and drove home alone.

I told myself, "Maybe she'll know me again tomorrow; maybe it's temporary."

But this encounter reminds me of the inevitable. If Molly's forgetting me is not now, it will be soon, and it hurts.

On the phone my friend Beth asked me if having Molly forget who I was worse than her dying. I replied, "I think dying will be worse. Now I can still see her face and feel some connection to whatever is left inside of the Molly I knew."

Her disease does not let me see inside her and Molly cannot communicate what is there. I am left to wonder.

For now, I feel abandoned. I don't like it. It is painful. Yet there is no place to run, no place to hide from the sadness.

What Do I Do Now? That is a very hard question to answer.

DEPRESSION

With Molly these days, things change day to day. Yesterday she "recognized" me. The previous two days she did not.

I put the recognized in quotes since I don't really know for sure what's going on inside her head. Sometimes she does give me a blank stare. Sometimes, she seems to prefer being with Mac.

When she does know me, we go out for a walk. We hold hands; we sing the songs she still knows over and over again. She is comfortable being with me. Sometimes she strokes my arm or leg in a loving way.

My moods go up and down. However, in the days since she first rejected my attentions and walked away with Mac, I have not spiraled down into depression. I've cried. I've grieved. Still it didn't seem like the sadness would last forever, like I couldn't stand to live with the emotion.

That's the way I felt in the days after I turned Molly over to the facility. Now that I'm faced with the sadness of losing Molly more and more, I'm less overwhelmed than I expected to be. I thought Molly's illness, decline, and death would lead to a breakdown.

My psychiatrist has diagnosed me as having major depression and explained it this way: I was abused and traumatized as a child. These experiences altered my brain chemistry. Once the changes in brain chemistry have been reinforced over time, they become permanent. Hence, I need anti-depressant medications to balance the chemical deficiencies in my brain.

While that seems logical and sensible, there may well be an alternative explanation: I had a rotten childhood. I learned I could get attention by telling sad stories about those times. The stories got more elaborate and more habitual. I would tell them to anyone who would listen: family members, work colleagues, Twelve Step group members, people at church, *therapists.*

Everyone sympathized with me. Everyone felt sorry for me. Everyone was concerned about me when I got depressed. I got a big payoff.

Molly's getting Alzheimer's and my exhausting myself caring for her gave me another opportunity to get people to feel sorry for me.

Since I stopped caregiving full time, I've had many other opportunities. The last time I saw my psychiatrist I was feeling good, making strides in self care and personal growth. I had completed my Fifth Step, was meditating every day, was progressing in A Course in Miracles. I had new friends, new activities. I was no longer isolated the way I was when Molly was home and I had to watch her every minute and keep her safe.

I said to my doctor, "I can't afford to see you for six months." She said, "You're doing so well right now, you don't need to see me for six months."

Maybe I also don't need people to feel sorry for me or Molly to get the attention and the help I do need.

SIMPLE PLEASURES

June 11, 2013

We had a very short spring this year. It snowed in April and into May. It's only early June, yet we are having hot summer weather: 97 degrees yesterday with 90 predicted for today.

Yesterday I took Molly to a wonderful homemade ice cream place in the same town as the facility.

Molly was fine about getting in the car, although when I fastened her seatbelt she got a little anxious. "And you?" she said. I assured her that I was indeed getting into the car with her. I fastened my seatbelt and showed her that I had mine on and she hers. She calmed down then. And off we went.

Since we had not been to this place for a couple of years I was off by a couple of blocks, but we found two girls on bikes to ask. Like everyone in town they knew how to get to Sweet Cow on a sunny day.

When we got inside, Molly was a little confused by the line—not too long considering the weather—she wanted to march right up to the front. Once we were in the line, it moved quickly and I ordered. "Two hot fudge sundaes. One with, let's see, oh yes, cookies and cream (for Molly) and do you have mocha or coffee?" "We have both." "Good." "One with coffee then." "Whipped cream? Almonds and pecans." "Everything with everything."

This last was Molly's approach to treats for the longest time. It applied, for example, to pie. When the waitress in a diner would ask, "You want ice cream with that, Hon?" Molly would reply with, "Yes, everything with everything."

Today Molly had a little trouble managing the whipped cream. It spilled onto the counter and the floor. But once she dug into the sundae, she was a happy camper. What could be better on a hot day! The waiter, proud that the ice cream, hot fudge, and whipped cream were made on site, told us that the ice cream was especially creamy. "It has a fat content of 12%," he bragged.

Molly gobbled up her portion and nodded enthusiastically when I opined, "It's really good, isn't it?" Simple pleasures. Molly relates strongly to what tastes good, especially sweet things. She is one of the few residents who have actually gained weight.

Her daughter, Dr. Nora, says, "What the heck. Just let her have what she wants and what tastes good to her. If she enjoys it, why not? It can't hurt at this point." So Molly gets everything with everything just the way she likes it.

I told Diane, who volunteers at the facility, where we were going. She put her hand on one hip and demanded, "Well, you'd better bring some back for us."

I did. One of the staff wrote "ice cream from Willem and Molly" on the top of the containers (one mint chocolate chip and the other vanilla). I later asked a care partner if she liked ice cream. I was prepared to tell her we had brought some, but the news had already spread. "I love ice cream. I heard you and Molly got some for us," she said with a smile.

Obviously Molly isn't the only one who enjoys simple pleasures.

LOVE REVISITED

I went hiking with my close friend, William, yesterday, and we had a long talk. The subject of love came up. We examined it for some time so the conversation got pretty philosophical.

William's bottom line went something like this: "Am I capable of loving someone else? If, when I ask that question, I get so frightened of the idea that the answer might be 'No,' then I can't really ask the question. My perspective is so skewed by the fear that I don't love anyone and can't love anyone that I can't really seek the true answer."

Shortly thereafter, I was describing my love for Molly, and, as I was getting into it, I slipped on a log and fell skinning my hand and elbow. We decided to just sit in the dirt for a little bit, and I talked about Molly as my soulmate and my partner.

Now that the Molly I knew is mostly gone, I have to love her in a new way. It is oversimplified, but it often seems perfectly accurate to say that I love her now as an adult loves a child.

If that is so, can I love again as I loved Molly before Alzheimer's? My Mother is still alive at 89. I might live another twenty-five years. It's a cliché to say, "Willem, Molly would not want you to be alone." But this one seems essentially, fundamentally true. I know that if our situations were reversed, I would want her to love and be loved.

Does this apply at all to Molly's friendship with Mac? Does she love him in any way that I would understand love. Maybe she does.

In the film *Away from Her,* the heroine who suffers from Alzheimer's gave signs of loving the man she met after she went into a facility. She forgot her husband and found someone else. I have used this story to help me with whatever jealousy I might feel towards Mac or Tom. Forgetting your spouse is a part of the disease. It's not personal.

What is love like for a person with Alzheimer's?   Molly still sometimes says, "I love you" to me and to others. I know she said it to Tom, because Sophie was a witness. Does she remember what love feels like? When she says "I love you" now, what does it mean to her?

The obvious question that arises is "Does she now 'love' Mac instead of me?"

This is an interesting question, but an irrelevant one. Sophie and I had discussed this when Molly was spending time with Tom. If Molly feels good now being with Mac and she gives and receives affection, then it is a good thing for her to have Mac in her life. She lives where he lives. She sees him every day. If she is happier when she is with him than when she is not, so be it.

As I write this, I am getting a knot in my stomach. That tells me that my mind has worked out all of this, but my heart is still struggling with the reality that Molly may love someone else, whatever that means for her at this point in her life.

And whatever it means for my seeking love elsewhere.

MOLLY DOESN'T EXIST

June 27, 2013

I had a car accident and totaled the car. Where I live, not having a car is not a practical option so I had to find another car.

I contacted my credit union and made an application over the phone. However, since I've been a full-time caregiver for years, I could not demonstrate enough income to qualify. The loan officer at the credit union was sympathetic, and we agreed to see if we could use Molly's Social Security and pension income to qualify.

It took a couple of days, but the answer was "Yes." Molly could qualify for a car loan. And I, as her Power of Attorney, could do all the paperwork. So far, so good.

I went used car shopping, never the most pleasant experience. I went through the usual routine with the salespeople. "The car you said you wanted to test drive isn't available yet. It's in the shop being prepped. But we have this other car that's the same model. Wouldn't you like to drive that one?" The substitute car shimmied at sixty miles an hour, and the engine raced every time I used first gear. No good.

I was, however, lucky enough to find a good dealer and a good car after three days of looking and test drives. I explained the situation with Molly and the power of attorney to the salesman and his manager. They called the credit union and determined that Molly was indeed qualified for an auto loan. Fine.

Then things started to go wrong, way wrong. State law requires that the dealer can only sell a vehicle to an individual with a valid driver's license. I had let Molly's driver's license lapse on her last birthday, since she wasn't driving and never would again. More discussion and negotiation. We could put both of our names on the sale documents and use my driver's license. OK. But that would mean an alternate ID for Molly. Did she have a passport? I said, "Sure," and drove home to find it.

When I got home, I went straight to the lockbox in the bedroom, opened it with the key, and extracted Molly's passport. I opened it only to read to my dismay that it had expired exactly one week earlier!

Molly had no valid ID. Molly didn't exist. Molly couldn't get a car loan. I had no income. I couldn't get a car loan either because I was a caregiver with no income. Shit.

In the end, I took out the last of my retirement nest egg and bought the car with cash three days later.

I created this story for myself. "This is the last car I will have to buy in my lifetime. I will drive it until I am 80. Then I will hand the keys to my grandson and say, 'Now you drive Papa.'"

Life is not just full of surprises. It is full of absurdities, and we are foolish if we think we have any control of what will happen.

DOES MOLLY RECOGNIZE ME OR NOT?

It's been a long time. I've adjusted to a new normal so often that I can't remember how many times it has changed.

The latest version of normal involves Molly's recognizing me or not. Wanting to be with me or not. It changes every day, and I don't know when I get there how she will behave.

"Do you want to go for a walk?" "No, I can't do that." Yes, sometimes she still speaks in complete sentences that make perfect sense. When she's like that, I used to try to get her attention and/or wait her out. Now I leave. I'll come back tomorrow or another day and see how she is that day.

One time last week, she didn't say anything or even make eye contact but she started humming "When You Wore a Tulip." That's one of our songs that we sing over and over again as we walk. I knew immediately that she was happy to see me and would go out for a walk with me.

Our walks are much shorter now. She seems to get confused more easily, and she points where she thinks we should be going. If we need to go another direction, I can tell her, "It's just down here, or over there. You'll see." She's still willing to take my hand and let me lead her.

Currently, we've gotten into a pattern of taking the short route to the coffee place. There is only one wide street to cross. When we get to the corner, Molly sees the sign and recognizes it.

When we get inside, it's mostly self-service. I can pour Molly decaf and add the milk and sugar myself. Then I get her a piece of pumpkin bread with chocolate chunks. Molly used to share this treat with me, but lately she eats it all herself.

Molly always seems interested in the fact that she is finished with her coffee and I'm still drinking mine. Sometimes, I'll pour a little bit out of my cup into hers. She likes that and smiles.

Most days, that's how it goes. An hour out of the facility, then back for music or bingo. When she does come with me, she is relaxed and comfortable with our set routine.

I am happy: I still get to sing with her and hold her hand.

MEDS A GIORNO

July 19, 2013

Molly was especially good today: alert and responsive. She called me "Papa" for the first time in weeks or perhaps months—I honestly can't remember.

She has not used my given name Willem more than once in over a year and a half. "Papa" is what the grandchildren call me, and so that's what Molly called me, too.

I was with a friend Jackie, who just retired as activity director at another facility for the elderly. Jackie had helped me choose Molly's current home. We visited it together, and she helped me decide.

Since Jackie had only seen Molly once since September when Molly went in, Jackie wanted to see how Molly was doing after nine months. Jackie was curious about how the place was operating.

We joined Molly as she ate lunch, and then the three of us took our regular walk to the coffee place. Then we came back to the facility for the afternoon's musical guests: this time it was three country and western singers, who did a little Frank Sinatra and Everly Brothers for variety.

I sang along to the songs I knew, and Molly joined in with me. She held my hand, and put her other hand on Jackie's knee. Molly was calm and content.

The only rough spot occurred earlier after lunch when the care partner was leading Molly to the bathroom. When I stopped at one of the lunch tables to talk to some of my favorite residents and help B.J. get the lid off her ice cream carton, Molly got cranky and resisted the care partner.

Afterwards, Jackie advised me, "You really shouldn't spend time with those other women when Molly is around. It really triggered her. After all, you're there for Molly. If she's out of the room, then it's all right to talk to them. But she can't handle it when you're not paying attention to her."

Message received. I had gotten in the habit of greeting the women at this particular table as we passed back and forth to Molly's room. I actually hadn't noticed that she got upset about my paying attention to someone else.

I think Jackie was right about what happened today. Molly was jealous. Hmmm. This started me wondering about my current status as compared to Mac.

In the car heading back, Jackie and I discussed another issue as well. Molly seemed much better today, and I noted that she had been out of meds for some time while we waited for the mail-order package to arrive. Could Molly, in fact, be better off without some of her meds?? This was definitely something to consider and discuss with her doctor.

The Director is very hawkish on meds. In particular, she had warned me that her experience showed that when patients went off their Alzheimer's drugs, they often declined and died shortly thereafter.

Then I was totally convinced.

Now I have my doubts.

DIGNITY OF CHOICE

Yesterday, when I got to the facility, Molly was already done with her lunch. I asked where she was, and one of the care partners pointed toward the courtyard. There she was, sitting outside with Harry. Harry is a relatively new resident. He is tall and thin and looks pretty old.

I went out to Molly and asked her if she'd like to take a walk. She said "No" and referred to Harry. She said something about him, "He . . ." and touched his leg. He smiled. I stared. Molly had made her choice for the moment, for the day.

I looked at her briefly, turned, and left, thinking "Harry is a new one. This isn't Mac whom she's been with for a long time. Will she/does she find any man to be with when I am not there? Does it matter who takes my place?"

That's her choice. There are few things left over which she has a choice. Others decide when she wakes up, what she wears, when she eats, what she eats, when she goes to the bathroom, when she takes a bath, when she goes for a walk, when she goes to bed.

I myself don't give her a lot of choices. When we go out for a walk together, I choose the songs we'll sing; I choose where we'll go and how long we'll be out; I pick our route going and coming back.

When we get to the coffee place, I pick her treat and prepare her decaf with milk, not cream, and unrefined sugar.   Sometimes she picks the table where we sit. When she finishes her coffee, I ask her, "Do you want some more?" I do abide by her, "Yes" or "No" answer.

Molly has so little control of her life that she is almost completely dependent.

I've thought a lot about how and when our relationship changed from adult-to-adult to adult-to-child. Even a small child gets to choose between peanut butter and jelly and grilled cheese, between milk and lemonade, between *Curious George* and *Richard Scary's Things That Go.*

But not Molly, not any more. One of the few choices she has left is "I want to be with Harry, not you. I want to stay here, not go out."

Who am I to take away that last shred of independence?

So I left. My departure was, I believe, a good choice for me.

And a good choice for Molly.

KEEP CHALLENGING

When I started writing this, I was convinced of many things, among them that there was nothing that would bring joy in my loneliness.   I also believed I had no idea how to take care of myself.

I can't say that I have learned to fully embrace change, but I certainly recognize now that change is the essence of life. For Molly and those she lives with, change manifests primarily in a gradual decline of functioning. For me, change has meant opportunities, especially time and energy for new interests and connections that lead to growth.

In particular, I now know sources of joy I had either not recognized or minimized. Playing Superman-to-the-rescue with my four-year-old grandson is, for example, extremely joyful every time.

I have also joined a hiking group and started to climb mountains with them. Yesterday, we climbed to the top of Mt. Audubon at 13,323 feet. The 13,000 level is significant to those of us who live in the Rocky Mountains. It's one step away from the ultimate thrill of summiting a 14'er. It was my first 13'er, and I was very happy with the achievement.

More importantly, it was an ecstatically beautiful day: perfect cool tempera- ture up high, glorious wildflowers blooming everywhere, stunning views of mountain peaks with their glaciers shining, radiant sky in a color of blue you can't see anywhere else.

This was coupled with good conversation up and down. Gary, one of the people I hiked with, is a personal trainer who works with people over 50 who have had a major injury. He himself has come back from a broken back.

Naturally, I asked him about Molly. "Molly lives in a place where everything is on one floor and she has lost some ability to do stairs. Is it important for her to keep doing stairs?" Gary's advice was specific and general, "She should do stairs whenever possible, and she should always be challenged to do as much walking and movement as possible."

I needed this input because I had been cutting back on the length and complexity of our daily outings as Molly has gotten more and more confused and uncomfortable. I, not unnaturally, assumed that she was better off with a short, easy, familiar route.

Gary reminded me that just as I am challenged by climbing mountains, Molly needs to be challenged as much as she can be. If she can walk three blocks, she can walk six blocks and the six-block walk is healthier regardless of whether or not she seems disoriented by a different path.

She can handle a little uncertainty, especially if she is holding my hand, and I can handle seeing her experience a little discomfort if it keeps her healthy longer.

There are different ways to respond to changes in life: keeping my curiosity going and my mind open to new perspectives helps immensely. This dog can still learn new tricks. For that I am most grateful, even joyful.

IT STILL HURTS

It still can hurt. Yesterday, I went to see Molly. It was a Sunday, so when I got to the facility they were doing the weekly prayer service. I sat in the back and waited.

I spotted Molly in the third row on a small loveseat (that's what you call the piece of furniture—not my fault). She was sitting with Mac. I saw her put her arm around him, and I got a little twinge of jealousy.

Later I went up to her and made eye contact.
WILLEM: Do you want to go out for a walk? (I pointed to the front door.)
MOLLY: No. (She inclined her head towards Mac.)
WILLEM: You just want to stay with him?
MOLLY: Yes.
WILLEM: Then I'll see you tomorrow.
MOLLY: Maybe.

I stood still, rather stunned. She was quite clear, apparently quite lucid. Definitely seeming to choose Mac over me at that moment and perhaps for the next day. And the day after that??

My next thought was to get out of there as quickly as possible. I used to try to wait her out, talk to some of the other residents for a while, and see if she'd change her mind. Not any more. Now when she says "No," I leave and wait for another day.

I was still upset when I got home. I wrote about the event in my Sixth Step notebook and called a Twelve Step contact to discuss how I was feeling.

The Sixth Step states "Became entirely ready to have God remove our defects of character." This Step in my program involves letting go of false ideas I have about myself, such as I am a failure. Part of the Sixth Step writing format is "Possibilities." Under that rubric we write what might have happened if we were not in the grips of the false self beliefs that come up out of habit.

In this case, my false self was telling me: "She's rejecting you. She doesn't care about you any more. She's abandoning you after thirty years." Telling myself this stuff obviously made me feel bad.

One of the alternative possibilities I discussed with my friend was taking a girlfriend with me to see Molly and saying, "You see. You have someone, and I have someone. We are all OK."

I do know full well that it is Alzheimer's that makes Molly cling to the nearest available male companion. One of the nurses says I should remember how Molly followed *me* around and see her actions as another version of the attachment behavior that comes with the disease. The nurse has a point.

I thought I had worked all of this out with Tom and Sophie months ago. Whatever makes Molly comfortable and content where she is is good.   If that's being with Tom, or Mac or Harry, so be it.

But yesterday, I was triggered again. I was surprised. Regardless of my level of familiarity and understanding, seeing her with someone else can still feel bad. It can still really hurt.

COMPANIONSHIP

August 5, 2013

I asked my friend Beatrice why she had gone onto an on-line dating site. She said simply, "Companionship" with just that edge to her voice suggesting that her answer should be obvious.

I was thinking about this a few weeks later when I was discussing dating with Peggy, another friend. She was talking about things she liked to do, such as go to art galleries on First Friday open houses. "It would be nice to have someone to go with."

When I am pondering my relationship with Molly now, I tend to think in terms of us as soulmates for thirty years and how that relationship has changed with her disease. We certainly cannot share time together the way we used to—bringing all of our intelligence, education, and life experience into play. "Remember what is was like when we first saw Chartres Cathedral together or when we heard Mozart played in Vienna?"

"Remember . . . ?" is never a good question to someone with Alzheimer's. Of course, she doesn't. The part of her brain where memories are stored is gone now.

Ah, but companionship—holding hands, singing a familiar song, sharing an ice cream sundae—that is still possible and precious.   Even the simple physical proximity of sitting in the driver and passenger seats in the car feels good to her, and to me.

I noticed this last night when I took her in the car to her son Chris's home for dinner. Her daughter Nora was visiting from New Orleans, and it was a special occasion.   Molly had a lovely time sitting around the dinner table with family and sharing a great meal.

When we got back to the facility, it was bedtime. After the care partner helped her into her pajamas, Molly lay down on her twin bed and I lay down beside her hoping she would go to sleep. She did almost immediately. When I left, she had the most peaceful look on her face.

I realized that companionship is still valuable to her. That is one of the reasons she finds a substitute "attachment" among the male residents when I am not around. Molly lived alone for about seven years after her divorce, but she has had me for a companion every day (minus a few business trips) for decades.

Having a companion (whoever he is) beside her feels comfortable, feels right. Molly knows that and does what she can to meet her need to "be with." The latter was a phrase we applied to our dogs and to ourselves: "I'm going to the store." "I'll come, too. I just want to be with."

"Being with" is still important.   Maybe more than ever.

PAUL, SANDY, AND ELLEN

August 18, 2013

"Where's Paul?" I asked one Monday morning. I hadn't seen him in a few days. "Oh, he passed last Thursday," replied the Assistant Activities Director. "He was joking with us on Tuesday; on Wednesday, he was in a coma; on Thursday, he died.   It was a good way to go. I wish it would be like that for everyone here. In fact, I hope when my time comes, it'll be just the same for me."

Before he died, Paul had gotten weaker and had been assigned briefly to the problem eaters table with Molly. He was seemed especially alert and sharp for someone with dementia. He had been a doctor, and I could tell somehow that he had been smart and good at medicine and at life. I would make eye contact with him and make some smart comment. He would wink in response. I could tell he always got the joke.

I liked him, damn it. I miss him. I miss seeing the spark of life that was still there in his bright eyes.

I also miss seeing him with Sandy. I was always on their side over the issue of their being a couple in the facility despite their respective dementias, and despite their families' objections.

The big surprise for me was how Sandy handled Paul's death. I expected some conventional grieving, that she would be sad and lonely without her companion. I might even see her crying.

But that's not how it played out. About a week after Paul's death, I noticed Sandy sitting in the front row for one of the musical guests. She was holding hands with Ellen. Over the next days and weeks, I observed them together all the time. Often holding hands.

Without missing a beat Sandy had replaced Paul with Ellen. Sandy, like Molly, is a person who needs a companion. If Paul was no longer available, then Ellen would do just fine.

I realized that I had projected my notions of a couple onto Paul and Sandy. I expected a couple to be one male and one female. I imagined that there was a romantic bond between them, and that they found each other attractive in a sexual way.

I had imagined the same thing about Molly and Mac and Molly and Tom. Yet what did I know about them or anyone else in their condition and situation? These are people whose brains have been damaged by illness. Their behavior is unpredictable and often strange. They live together in a locked facility.

How could I possibly know what Sandy felt for Paul or vice versa? I couldn't, so I relied on stereotypes drawn from people who don't have Alzheimer's. If I saw them holding hands and smiling at each other, I made assumptions about their feelings.

So I was surprised when Ellen became Sandy's new special friend. Silly me.

DIVERSITY AND NOT AS BAD AS

Since I am a white male, it may seem a little odd that I have been involved in diversity programs, even as a co-facilitator. My qualifier, such as it was, was poverty. When my family moved to the suburbs of Chicago in the 1950s, there were no blacks or Hispanics or Jews or open gays in our town of 10,000. The local bullies targeted me and some of my siblings as the "other"—the poor kids with holes in their shoes and too many children in their house.

In any case, I grew up with a strong sense of rooting for the underdog and favoring minorities and oppressed groups. I was an impressionable twelve-year-old when Kennedy became the first Catholic elected president. My parents were into civil rights for blacks early on. My father, for example, created quite a stir when he cast a black woman to play Juliet opposite a white Romeo in the early 1960s. I have nine sisters and a Mother: in the 1970s I became a feminist and subscriber to *Ms. Magazine.*

Later I joined my work colleague and friend Angelo Lewis who is black and Filipino when he founded the Diversity Table discussion series at Princeton University. This led to Angelo's co-founding the Diversity and Spirituality Network, which included diversity trainers who worked with government agencies in Washington. Angelo and I even did some diversity training together.

Thus I have some personal and professional perspective on diversity issues. Alzheimer's is, of course, an "equal opportunity" disease: it affects all people regardless of race, class, gender, sexual orientation, or ethnicity. Yet, in Molly's facility, the resident population is all white and about two-to-one female. (This is purely economic and not a symptom of discrimination.) The staff, especially the front-line caregivers are, on the other hand, completely diverse, including blacks, Hispanics, Asians, and probably some gays.

The situation seems at first glance to be very 1950s old-fashioned. Here's a black woman bathing an elderly white woman who can afford to pay for her services. The reality is much more positive. The institution reflects the more inclusive attitudes of a post-"I Have a Dream," post-feminist movement society. The community is very open, tolerant, and varied, and there is no evidence whatever of discrimination in hiring or promotion.

Yet, it is striking to sit in the dining area at mealtime and look around at all of the white, middle-and upper-class folks who live there. Obviously they all got there because of The Disease, some form of dementia, mostly Alzheimer's. On the surface, the resident population is primarily little old ladies with curly perms who are having trouble keeping track of their walkers.

Having been around this small group of fifty-two people for many months, I now see quite a bit of diversity: physical, emotional, and behavioral. Some of the patients are in wheelchairs and/or need oxygen tanks to breathe. Some are also victims of osteoarthritis and are permanently hunched over. Some have symptoms of other diseases, such as Parkinson's. Some participate in activities while others spend most of the day asleep in the common areas. Some are always cheerful and smiling while others can be continually hostile and confrontational.

I find that my reactions and responses to the residents fall into two main categories. First, and foremost, I see the decline in physical and mental capabilities and the behavioral changes that indicate the progression of their dementia. This elicits mostly fear and sadness—for the residents and for Molly.

Inevitably, I also compare Molly's condition with that of others, usually in an attempt at reassuring myself. "Well, Molly is having more trouble walking, but at least she's not helpless in a wheelchair like Genevieve." "Molly often spills her food on her clothing, but she doesn't make nearly as much of a mess as Doc." "Molly may withdraw and space out, but at least she's not hostile to everyone like Mavis."

It may be pretty silly exercise, but, at least temporarily, it feels good to believe that Molly is "better" than someone who is clearly worse off. It means she's not so ill; she's not in obvious pain; she's not too near death. Such comparisons and distinctions are designed to keep the truly unpleasant thoughts and feelings at bay. I guess that denial is OK for me right now.

Molly will get sicker and more disabled, and she will die.   I will grieve each loss as it comes.   But, maybe, not today.   Because, just for today, she's not as bad as . . .

I CRIED TODAY

September 7, 2013

I cried today.   At the facility.   In front of Molly although she didn't seem to notice.   This is something I often told myself I would never do.

A year ago on admitting day, I sobbed bitterly in the parking lot outside, but I had never wept where Molly or any other resident or staff member could see me.

How did it happen?   Immediately beforehand, Sally had told me, "My Mom is in hospice now. . . . About three months.   I will take her home at some point."   Her Mom is B.J., my favorite resident.

I first met B.J. at the fall dance last year.   She was sitting across the room with Mary, another of her daughters, and her grandson Matthew.   Her blue eyes shone, sparkled, glowed with life and spirit.

Since that first meeting, I have made eye contact with B.J. whenever I could. I have joked and flirted with her, helped her take the top off her ice cream cup, commented often on the weather outside, and sung "When You Wore a Tulip" for her.

B.J. sits at the head of the ladies table with a group that has been regular for most of the last year.   I learned their names so I could greet them all without seeming to favor B.J.   But she was and is my favorite.

Moreover, Sally is my favorite visiting relative.   Sally always smiles and keeps her energy up.   I cannot imagine ever seeing her cry in public.   Today, she bustled about the dining room serving coffee and tea to the ladies.

Outwardly, Sally seems unphased by B.J.'s decline, but the fact that she couldn't sit still at lunch was telling.

Today was a Friday, so we had live music. Tony Zain offered us pretty acceptable imitations of Nat King Cole, Tony Bennett, Andy Williams, and Neil Diamond.   I sang along while Molly dozed a little and sang a little herself.

Where I was sitting, B.J. and Sally were on my left and Molly on my right. The news that B.J. had only a few months to live was sinking in when Tony launched into "Just the Way You Are" by Billy Joel.

Everything in the song seemed to refer to me and Molly and her Alzheimer's: "I wouldn't leave you in times of trouble. We never could have come this far. I took the good times, I'll take the bad times. I'll take you just the way you are." By the end of the fourth verse, where he sings "I just want some- one that I can talk to. I love you just the way you are," tears were running down my face. Sometimes I desperately miss the Molly I could talk to.

I glanced at Sally. She was looking straight ahead, giving me space to grieve privately.

As I left out the back door, Sally was right behind me. She spoke to me about the "journey" towards death that she was embarking on with her Mom.

I took a chance, and I said, "You must have seen me crying."   "Yes," Sally replied "'I love you just the way you are' is your new theme song." I know I nodded, but I can't remember coming up with a reply. Then Sally said, "I love you, Willem, just the way you are." "Thank you, Sally."

We got into our cars and drove our separate ways. I felt much better. I am not alone in my loss or in my grieving.

EMBARRASSING

This is embarrassing. For two days, Molly didn't recognize me and I went off the deep end.

I took a break until the end of the week and then went back to see her. She recognized me again.   So much for "the end" I feared and imagined. The fear is real. Alzheimer's only progresses in one direction: downhill.

Imagining what the future will bring is another story. It's like everything else in life. One day at a time. "Most of the things you worry about never actually happen." Can't remember where I read that, but it is true.

I'm not sure anymore if it makes sense to label Molly's behavior as another "new normal." It changes all the time. My role is to accept whatever happens or doesn't happen on any given day. Molly may recognize me or not; Molly may be willing to go for a walk with me or not. That's the disease.

How I respond is up to me. It does seem to help to have a strategy, and developing one has taken much trial and error over time. If Molly doesn't want to go out, I just leave and come back another day.

The same basic principle applies to Molly's decline and the way I view the losses I see. She forgets more and more. She gets tired more easily. She has more trouble with eating: she uses utensils less and less and fingers more and more.

I observe; I notice; I grieve; and, when I am in a good place, I accept.

Recently, the lyrics to the Billy Joel song "I love you just the way you are" made me weep uncontrollably. Now that sentiment seems more like a practical approach to life on life's terms.

I had to learn—sometimes the hard way—that there are "things I cannot change." I know where I read that. It is in the first line of the Serenity Prayer: "God, grant me the serenity to accept the things I cannot change, courage to change the things I can, and wisdom to know the difference."

I am older and much, much wiser. I know that the journey and the lessons continue and will continue until the end of Molly's lifetime and mine. And, who knows, perhaps even beyond?

BOTH/AND

November 29, 2013

It is four days since Thanksgiving. When I took Molly to her son Chris's home we had a full Thanksgiving meal: I made the stuffing and the gravy; Molly's grandson Matthew made the cranberry sauce; Molly's daughter-in-law Beth made the sweet potatoes; and Chris made the pumpkin pies. The meal was delicious, and Molly enjoyed every bit of it.

She, however, signaled that she was finished by pouring her sparkling apple juice onto her dinner plate. I projected my perception onto her and determined that she was tired and had had as much stimulation as she could handle. Molly needed to go "home" and rest where everything is familiar and routine. I took her back to the facility, where they were serving a dinner she was too full to eat.

When I left her, I felt a deep and widespread sadness. Part of me still wishes she were as she was before: that she could experience the excitement of anticipating the holiday, feel the joy of being with loving family, and keep the day in her memory.

I know she cannot. Most of the time I accept this new normal. It was wonderful that she could be with us for a few hours and enjoy the simple pleasure of eating good food with loving people around her.

Yet my grieving process continues. Some of the intense emotions that have arisen in the past year have lessened. I was still sad.

I felt like going home and taking a nap and starting the day over: I had another party to go to at Karl and Beth's with many of my closest friends. I didn't want to feel the sadness that arises from knowing that Molly will never get any better. Perhaps this is her last Thanksgiving outside a facility.

Then I thought, "This sadness is real. You must face it and go through it. Shutting down is not going to help." I decided to go home, pick up my pie, and go to be with my friends. No Molly, but . . .

It took several hours, but by the end of the evening I was having a good time. I wrote a thank you note to hostess Beth, and she replied, "You are so welcome. It was fun for me for you to be there, especially participating in Apples to Apples [the game we played]. When you enjoy yourself, it's contagious. Thanks for being here. You were a great addition. Dear Molly, she continues to be known and loved, especially by you."

With Molly and Alzheimer's, love and grief go hand-in-hand. That is reality. Much of the time, I believe I have reached the acceptance phase of the grieving process, but it is never completely finished. Sometimes I cycle back to anger or sadness.

But I do have choices now. I am not overwhelmed when strong emotions arise. I have a life. I have loving family and friends. I can feel uncomfortable emotions and still be OK.

In fact, I can feel sadness *and* happiness. It is, as Buddhist philosophy says, not either/or but rather both/and.

PAIN AND GRIEVING

"When the student is ready, the teacher will appear." I have heard this many times and accept it as fundamentally true. Still I didn't realize that the teacher might appear before the student was ready and go away and come back again.

Two days ago as I was walking past a bookcase in my living room, I stopped to look at the self-help and recovery books on the shelf. I recognized John Bradshaw's book with its bright red cover. Several books over was a nondescript paperback with a puzzling title *Legacy of the Heart: The Spiritual Advantages of a Painful Childhood* by Wayne Muller. "Advantages? What the heck was that about?"

I opened the book. It was, indeed my book; it had my notes in the margins. It also had a receipt—now faded but still legible—that showed when I had bought it: August 9, 1994. Over nineteen years ago! At that time, I had read—judging by the margin notes—the first five chapters. So, out of curiosity, I started to read Chapter Six.

It was a revelation. It began by saying that when we were hurt in childhood, we thought our wounds, our brokenness, made us special. We were also especially sensitive to the sufferings of others and believed we had special gifts to comfort and heal them. "We learned to see ourselves as set apart from the rest of the world, both by the unique gifts and by the terrible sufferings that were given to us."

In fact, our sufferings did not really make us special in an isolated way. Instead they made us like everyone else because all people suffer pain. If we are willing and able to face our own pain, then "we claim kinship in a new family—a broad and rich family of everyone who has ever rejoiced and who has ever suffered, who have sung and grieved just as we have done."

This last year with Molly and her Alzheimer's has given me the opportunity to feel my pain and to grieve.

I tried other strategies: I tried denial. I tried distraction. I tried blaming God. I tried fighting everyone as an advocate for Molly's care. I tried programs of spiritual growth.

Yet I was still sad. I still mourned Molly's losses and my losses. I still felt miserable with self-pity: Why was this happening? How could life and God and the Universe be so unfair?

More importantly I also wrote these pieces, and I committed myself to being as honest about my experiences as I could be at any given time. That would be how I believed I could help others who went through the same difficulties.

So the sadness arose, and I would write about it, crying over my keyboard. Then finally I cried at the facility in front of Molly and the other residents and the staff.

I still have more grieving to do. Molly is alive and healthy. When her body goes into its final decline and she dies, the pain may be overwhelming for a time. But I know now—know deeply—that I can face that pain and survive.

I will be just like all the others, some of whom I now know as friends and helpers on the journey of grief and many more whom I will never know personally but who have lost a mother or a father or a spouse or a child. I grieve with them all.

Now I am most grateful to really understand that I am not alone.

This piece is dedicated to Sally and Leslie.

WRITE WHEN YOU HAVE SOMETHING TO SAY

I thought I was finished with this part of the grieving process and this part of my writing about it.

Then today I went to visit Molly. She was sitting on a sofa in the lounge staring into space. When I got her attention, she smiled and said "Hi." She stood up. I gestured for her to come with me, and she said, "No, I can't do that."

I whispered in her ear one of our code phrases "Out and about," and I did get her to follow me into the lobby and to the entrance door. I punched in the door lock code and opened the door for her. Again, "No, I can't do that."

She turned and walked quickly away from me towards the other wing of the building. A nurse followed her and tried to persuade her to go out with me. Failing, the nurse returned and gave me a shrug. I said, "I'll try again tomorrow" and left.

The reason I am writing this is that, as I was going, I felt a knot in my stomach. "That's where anxiety lodges," I thought.

So what am I afraid of at this point, having been through the new normal of Molly's not recognizing me, Molly wanting to be with Mac, etc. for months now?

Is it still the basic fear of abandonment? Is it my identity/ego? If Molly, my best friend, my partner, my lover, my wife for thirty years says "No" to me, does that mean I am less than? Or, even, worthless?

I am crying now so I guess I have touched some still sensitive, grieving place.

If I have lost her, have I lost myself?

Not really. I know that now. I am who I am not because I love Molly and she loves me and I take care of her and advocate for her and visit her and sing with her and feed her sweets. I am not half of Molly and Willem. I am a human being on my own terms.

So why the feeling of sadness beneath the fear of abandonment? How long will I grieve this loss of our special relationship? How long will I grieve the loss of her inevitable death?

I don't know; I can't know until I see it all behind me with the 20/20 vision of hindsight.

But I do know that today I needed to write this.

MOLLY CHANGES AGAIN

December 2, 2013

I thought I was OK. I had adjusted to the new normal in which Molly recognizes me most days and some days does not, adjusted to seeing her with other men and her preferring their company to mine.

But I was not OK when she suddenly changed towards me in a more dramatic way. I went to visit at lunchtime as usual. I pulled up a chair and sat next to her. She stared at me. I cut up her food as I have done many, many times. She moved the plate away from me and then moved her coffee cup and water and juice glasses.

I thought, "She seems to think I am going to take her food. . . . Maybe she is just finished." I said, "You could share it with me." "No, I can't do that." I pierced a piece of chicken with her fork and offered it to her. "Don't do that," she said.

It was becoming clear that she didn't recognize me, but it was more than confusion: she was seeing me as a stranger and a threat.

Oh, my God, this is it. This is what I have been dreading.

I left the table and went into the serving room with a staff member I know well. "I need a hug, and I am going to cry." I cried. Susan held me.

I went back to the table to try one more time. I started to sit next to Molly. "Don't come here," she said. She turned her back on me and started to talk to the woman next to her. I got up and left the room.

She had walked away before but she had never aggressively sent me away.

It hurt. It hurt like Hell.

Once outside, I called my friend Beth and cried. She talked me down with her Buddhist-derived wisdom. We can accept reality or we can fight it. When we accept it, we can find peace. When we fight it, we suffer.

I am back to grieving big time, and acceptance comes *after* denial, anger, negotiation, and sadness. I am not at acceptance yet, not even close. This is too painful. It will take time.

I thought, after a year, that I had reached acceptance. Molly has Alzheimer's. It is a powerful disease. It controls her. Molly is not trying to hurt me. The part of her brain that remembered me and knew who I was is damaged and, now, maybe gone forever.

There is nothing I can do about it. She is sick, and there is no cure.

Alzheimer's is a terrible disease. Molly will not survive it. Yet she does not feel pain.

I feel the pain of her losses and mine, but I will survive. Acceptance will come eventually. After all, it's the disease that makes Molly forget not Molly herself.

It is all very confusing.

THE LIGHT IN HER EYES

Dec 9, 2013

Laurinda, my friend from A Course in Miracles wrote to me: *"Tonight, when I was describing the movie about Amma, the hugging woman . . . what moved me were the people she hugged. She gave them hope. She brought out their vulnerability. They wanted a profound connection. They were SO beautiful. The movie was slow and my heart opened and I had this experience of loving people, of feeling just a little bit closer to being less scared and more certain we are all one.*

I wonder if you have had a similar experience in taking care of Molly? I mean, you must have had to slow down as she slowed down. And you have had to look past all the Alzheimer's to find her. And the moments you do find her, you look at her and say, 'Here you are, my beautiful wife.' And you are totally in the present moment, and your heart is open."

I replied: *"The pace of life and all activities is much slower with Molly now. And I am much more patient with adjusting to her pace/rhythm. I see her beauty sometimes when she smiles at me and I see the light in her eyes. (I am crying now.)*

She used to say, 'I love you.' Now it is only the eyes.

Sometimes, too, she will laugh at an inside joke we still share somehow, or a phrase we used. When we leave the building to go for a walk, I will whisper in her ear, "Let's go out and about." I do it with a Scottish accent so it sounds like oot and aboot. She likes that and smiles and laughs.

We used to have three songs we sang as we walked around the neighborhood where she lives. We are down to one: When You Wore a Tulip. She hums the tune sometimes when she sees me, and I start to sing the words. Then, she remembers some of it and sings along as best she can. She is usually with me by the last line: 'Your lips were sweeter than julep when you wore a tulip and I wore a big red rose.'"

Yesterday at Molly's facility, there was a tea party for Christmas, and all of the residents had their pictures taken with Santa. One of the caregivers came by our table and asked Molly to smile. She did. It was lovely.

When we had the picture taken, Santa had us say "Cookie," and Molly smiled beautifully.

The picture is precious, a reminder that, yes, my beautiful wife is still here.

SURRENDER

January 2, 2014

I have never given up, but I must surrender.

Surrender to the inevitable. Alzheimer's is terminal, incurable, and untreatable. If something else doesn't kill her first, Molly will die from it. Possibly much sooner than I expected.

The soon was something I never quite believed till now. "Molly is strong," I would say. "She has no heart trouble, no diabetes. She will live a long time."

Apparently, not so. The disease has been exercising a slow decline over the course of years. Now, the pace has accelerated: the decline is rapid. Soon, too soon.

I had been away for Christmas. I went to see my daughter and son-in-law and new grandchild on the coast of New Jersey. Sophia is 10 ½ months old. I got to be with her, to play with her, at her first Christmas. That was so joyful as to require different words to express my feelings. It was "blissful." With Sophia in my arms, I was as happy as a person can be.

While I was gone, I got phone calls telling me that Molly was having a series of seizures.

And that she had developed an upper respiratory infection that might be pneumonia.

The first time I saw Molly after I returned, her son Chris was there, too. I was holding Molly's hand and asked Chris to go and speak with the nurse about Molly's condition.

When Chris came back, he asked me to go to another room so we could speak privately.

He told me that the nurse had said Molly's condition was very bad. The nurse had suggested that we consider taking Molly off her antibiotics and letting the pneumonia take its course BECAUSE PNEUMONIA WAS AN EASY WAY TO PASS.

"Oh, my God," I cried out, and then I wept.

Molly was going to die, might even be dying. I was in shock. "How could this be? When I left, she was fine. She was walking to the coffee bar and singing Christmas carols with the Girl Scouts."

The disease had passed some tipping point. Seizures are a symptom of late stage Alzheimer's in 10-20% of cases. Molly had had a few before, one grand mal years earlier that put her in the emergency room. Now they were coming in bunches, sometimes continuously with one limb in spasm over and over again.

After I cried and after Chris left, I called A Course in Miracles friend. We had set a time to have coffee after my visit. She said, " I'm not sure we should meet today. I am going through a stressful time with my daughter, and I don't feel very stable." "Well, I am in a place where I need to receive today. If you can't give today, then we can reschedule." She called back in half an hour to say she could offer support. We went for a walk which helped a lot.

Later I called Jackie for more support. Jackie has worked as a social worker and activities director in many senior care places. She volunteered to go with me, and we visited Molly and held her hands until she fell peacefully asleep.

Molly even said to Jackie, "It's all good."

I don't feel that way, but it is reality. The next day Molly was admitted to hospice. The only way to qualify for hospice care is for two doctors to determine that you are in the last six months of life.

I am still in shock, still in disbelief, still in denial. Molly is dying.

Too soon, too soon.

ACCELERATED DECLINE

One of the remarkable things about my lifetime has been the progress in treating illness and disease. When I was a child, one still saw people in braces from polio. Then the vaccine was developed, and we were spared the pain of polio.

When I was young, cancer was the big C. A diagnosis of cancer was a death sentence. My grandfather died so quickly from cancer that my mother was as shocked as if he had had a heart attack. Now there are many varieties of cancer treatment, and, for most patients, survival is not only possible but probable.

Not so with Alzheimer's. Molly is going to die from Alzheimer's.

Her symptoms are getting worse. Three weeks ago she experienced a perfect storm of a series of seizures, a chest infection, and constipation that weakened her to near death. The hospice nurse told me that after such a crisis she might well improve, but that she would be weaker, less healthy.

Molly bounced back after her crisis; it was a very loud false alarm. Molly is physically much stronger than the staff nurse or I believed.

However, Molly has not returned to where she was before Christmas. Yesterday I observed a number of disturbing symptoms: she has more trouble eating, more trouble with chewing and so on; she has a shorter attention span; she is more physically disabled—she has more difficulty getting out of a chair, walking, or climbing even a small flight of stairs. She tires more easily. She is more confused and uncertain.

I took her for our regular walk yesterday: two blocks to Paul's Coffee and back. On the way there, her pace was very slow and unsteady. When we got to the intersection where we used to cross at the red light, she couldn't understand that the cars would stop and she wouldn't move. I had to take her to the middle of the block and wait until no traffic was coming. Then, if I held her and talked reassuringly, she could get across.

When we got to the coffee place, she was clearly tired out, and she dozed in her chair before she drank her decaf with milk and sugar. She was also remarkably disinterested in her favorite treat: pumpkin bread with chocolate chunks.

She did rally somewhat on the way back, her stride more confident and "normal."

However, she was much less animated than usual during the Sunday service, singing some of the hymns with enthusiasm as before but spacing out at other times.

I had to concede that Molly is worse than a few weeks age, that her decline has accelerated as the hospice nurse predicted, that she is not going to return to her pre-crisis baseline.

I don't like any of this. It is such a terrible disease, relentless and heartbreaking.

Yet, we did have precious moments when she made definite eye contact and recognized me, when she smiled at me and kissed me, when we sang together as we walked. I am grateful for every one.

Part Three: The Long Road

SECOND COMING OF THE ANGEL SARAH

January 20, 2014

How many angels are named Sarah? I wrote a longtime ago about one Sarah who helped me search for Molly when she wandered away from a restaurant. That Sarah appeared and disappeared almost magically.

Today Molly fell and hit her head on a doorframe splitting her forehead open. The wound required eleven stitches.

There we were at the urgent care facility. Molly was being prepped for the stitches to be done by the doctor. The procedure required numbing the area, which meant sticking a large needle into Molly's forehead multiple times.

I was sitting on the edge of the bed holding Molly's hand. The doctor asked if I would hold both of Molly's hands out of the way while she administered the medication.

I had no idea what I was facing. Molly could not understand our telling her that we were helping her and that the "sting" was necessary.

She screamed in pain each time the needle went in. She writhed and tried to escape. I held her, and I wept. She even called me by the pet name "Wuggie," which I thought she had forgotten. She wanted me to stop the pain. I couldn't. It was terrible.

Later while the doctor stitched up the wound, Molly reacted to the needle, and the doctor gave her another needle of numbing fluid. By then, I was numb myself. I couldn't believe this was happening.

At this low point, Sarah appeared. This angel I had already met. This Sarah is a leader of the Buddhist sangha I attend every other Tuesday. I have sat with her in meditation dozens of times. We have spoken occasionally, and Sarah has participated in the sangha's prayer for our son D.J. after he was stabbed.

Amazingly, here she was, coming in to do Molly's wound care and custom cut her bandages and to be present with me in a spiritual way that was calming and reassuring.

Immediately the energy in the room shifted. I knew I was OK. I knew Molly was OK.

This Sarah is tall and blonde and beautiful on the outside. She is, no doubt, even more beautiful inside.

There was an angel in one of my dreams who looked quite different and whom I nicknamed Abigail. Perhaps if I dream of her again, I should change her name.

"Sarah" sounds right.

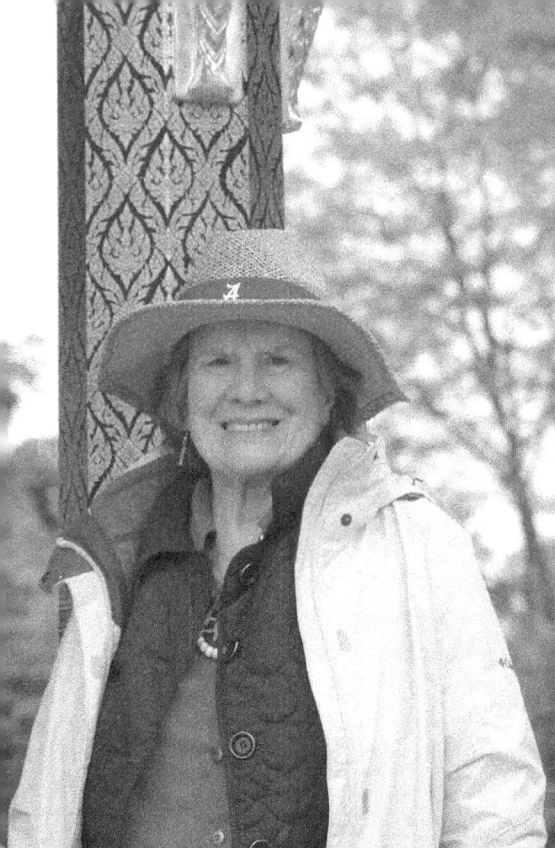

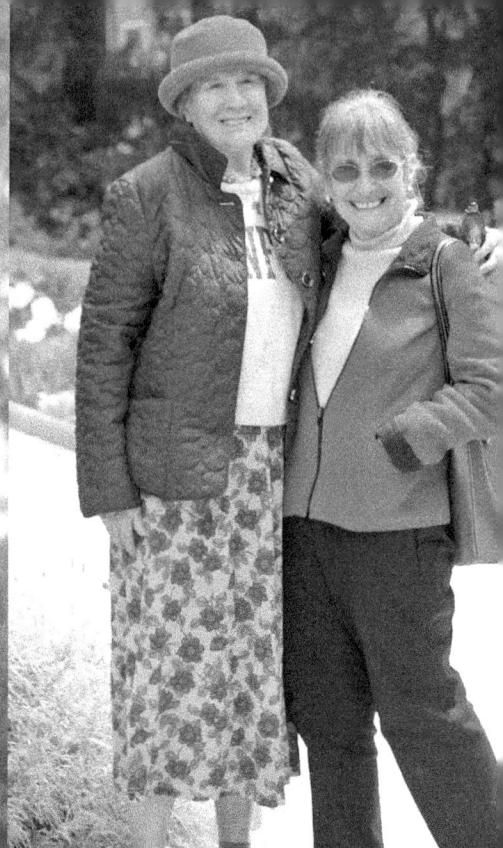

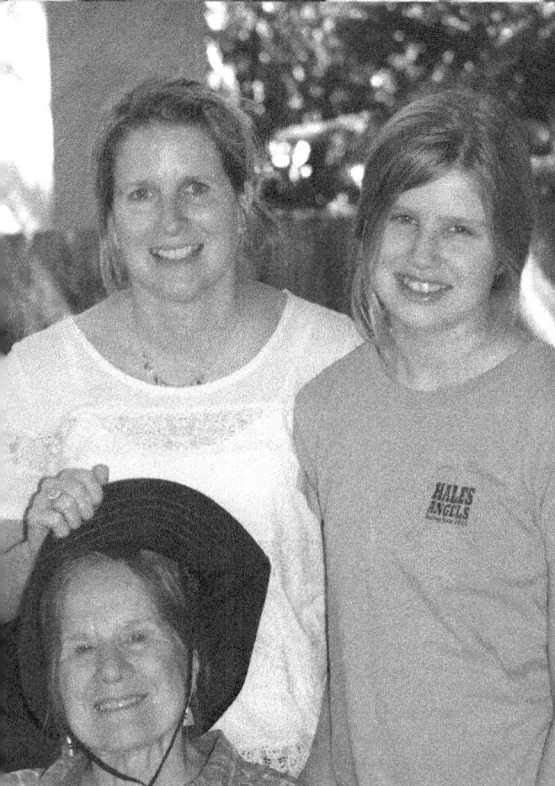

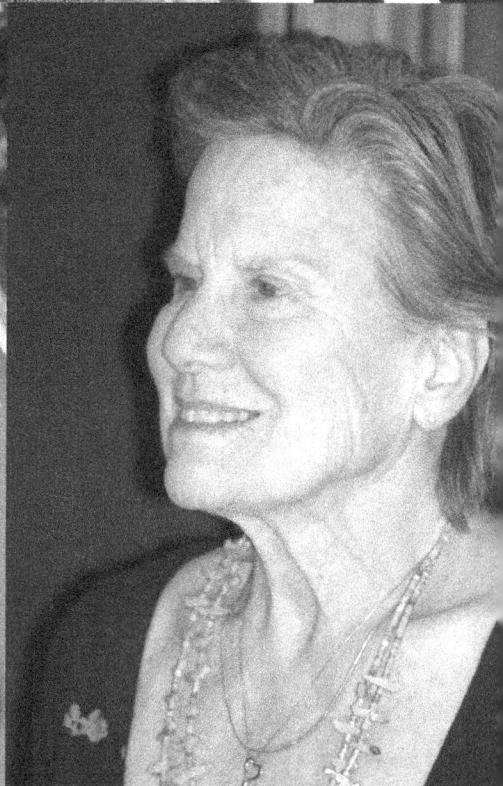

Molly at the botanic gardens in Madison, Wisconsin; Molly with friend of 50 years Alicia Ostriker, Princeton, New Jersey. Molly with Nora and granddaughter Emma; Molly wearing her favorite necklace of turquoise birds.

NOT SPECIAL

I grew up the oldest of fourteen children. We were poor. During my first six years of education, I went to a different school every year because we were always behind on the rent and forced to move.

Later we moved to an all-white, middle-class suburb. There, we lived in a three-bedroom, one-bath house that was a converted summer home with the last coal furnace in the county. The kids in our neighborhood and at school teased me and beat me up. I went to the hospital with concussions three times.

My Mother told us that despite our being poor we were special because we were smart and talented and kind. I thought I was special because I was shy and fearful from being different and getting beaten up.

Are you, dear reader, feeling sorry for me yet? I did. I felt sorry for myself for decades and decades. It seemed to be a good strategy. People felt pity for me. I got attention, comfort, and affection. I came to believe it was the only way I could be loved.

I now see how dysfunctional that was.

When I left the clinic last week after Molly's treatment for her head wound, I thought I was special again because something really bad had happened to me and someone I care about. I wasn't so special. One of the first people I told my story to was Molly's hospice nurse who said she had had the same experience going to the doctor with her Down's Syndrome child. Not special, but the same.

The nurse didn't automatically feel sorry for me because she's healthier than that. She did comfort me, but in solidarity not pity. Hmmm.

I have had many reactions to this writing: "honest," "true," "moving," "inspiring." Only once did a good friend have the temerity to say, "When I read this, I felt sorry for you, and I don't think that is what you are trying to do."

She was right: it is not at all my intention this time. I want the book to be helpful, informative, inspiring, but not pity inducing.

I am special, not because Molly has Alzheimer's and the Universe is unfair to make her and me suffer. If I am special, it is only because I am the same as every caregiver who loves someone with a terminal, incurable, untreatable disease. We all feel the same shocks, the same losses, the same guilt, the same confusion, the same frustration.

I happen to be able to write about it. That's all.

Many people say, "I can't imagine how it must be for you." I *can* imagine how it is for all of the family members and friends I have met over the days and months. We share the same ups and downs, the same fears, the same uncertainties.

I have learned that the pain and suffering of life are about *we* not I. That understanding is special.

CAREGIVING 501: ADVANCED COURSE

I developed patience because I had to. The "care partners" who work where Molly lives chose to master the practice of patience. Sure, it is a job requirement. Still I believe their patience reflects their essential goodness, generosity, and compassion.

No matter what Molly's behavior over the years, the care partners always said to me. "I like Molly. We all love Molly."

Molly is, indeed, very lovable almost all the time. She looks good. She smiles often. When she was still communicating with words, she said "Thank you." So it's not surprising that she should be a staff favorite. There are others who speak and behave in angry, irritable, and, even, hostile ways most of the time.

That's only half the picture at best. These care partners are extraordinary people. They really do care, really do go the extra mile, really do strive to get to know and to help their charges in every way they can.

I like to go to visit Molly during lunchtime. It's when all of the residents on her side of the building gather in one place. It's when I can talk to the care partners as they serve the meal and feed people and clean up.

Lunchtimes are often an opportunity for social interaction, especially with Tom and Sophie and with B.J. and her daughter Sally. It has been a time of closeness when Molly needed help and I started to feed her.

I like feeding Molly. Sometimes, I convince myself that I am still needed, that if I wasn't feeding her she wouldn't get enough protein or enough vegetables. That I know full well is all a fantasy in my own head.

I have watched the care partners feed her. They are just as attentive, just as careful, just as aware as I—probably more so. For one thing, I am only around for three or four meals a week, while they feed Molly the other seventeen or eighteen. They're the ones who tell me, "She ate her whole breakfast this morning. 100%." I wasn't there at 8:00 a.m. They were.

The same is true regarding other aspects of Molly's physical well-being. If Molly falls, one of them helps her up. If Molly has trouble sleeping and wanders into the common area, one of them puts a blanket on her in the armchair. When Molly seems cold, one of them gets her a sweatshirt.

It is true that Molly's particular facility has a small population of only fifty-two and a very good staff-to-patient ratio. I still find the care partners concern and affection for Molly beyond my hopes and expectations.

These are good people. They love their work, and they do it well day in and day out. Molly is in good hands. I am very grateful.

30TH ANNIVERSARY

Yesterday, February 10, 2014, was Molly's and my 30th wedding anniversary.

I have been saying for some time that I wanted to do something to celebrate and mark the day even though Molly would not know what was going on.

I actually planned a family lunch for last Saturday, but the winter weather and work schedules forced us to postpone two weeks. "Molly will not know the difference," I said, and it is true.

People always ask me now, "Does she recognize you?" It is not, as they expect, a yes or no question anymore. It is much more, "*How* does she recognize you? How does she react to your presence? How does she act when you are with her?"

She "recognizes" me when she starts humming the melody of a song we have sung together many times. She recognizes me when she smiles. She recognizes me when she clings to me as we cross the street watching out for traffic.

She recognized me when she was in pain and fear in the urgent care clinic and she called me by my pet name.

Last night I went to see Molly at dinnertime. I fed her dinner and dessert. Then she started to fall asleep in her chair so I escorted her over to a sofa near the fireplace. I sat on the floor next to her and put my head on her knee.

She recognized me by stroking my hair. I cried, because I miss her tender touch so much.

Did Molly know this was a special day for me and for her? No, I don't think so. Did she acknowledge, in the way she still could, the bond that has grown over the last three decades? Yes, yes, yes.

Later I texted Molly's daughter Nora about my visit with her Mom. She sent me back a photo of us on one of our visits to New Orleans. We both looked happy, relaxed, young, and healthy. It was a lovely reminder of good times—so many good times over so many years in so many places.

So, like the Buddhists, who see life in terms of both/and rather than either/or, I came away from this anniversary with joy and sadness, both/and. Not one or the other. Yes, this day was sad, but it was also blissful to feel her hand on my hair in a gesture of love.

Our love is different now. Our love will never be the same as it was before, but just because it is different does not make our love any less true.

Happy Anniversary, Molly. I love you.

TOOLS FOR SELF-CARE II

March 14, 2014

Much as I try to stay in the present moment, there are occasions when the passage of time seems all too apparent.

It has been one and one half years since Molly went into the memory-care facility. She's been there for two Christmases, one landmark birthday (her 75th), our thirtieth anniversary, the birth of her eleventh grandchild. Time has passed.

There is definitely a time before September 10, 2012, and after. Since Molly entered the facility, she has changed, and so have I. I've already experienced "anticipatory grief" in all five stages. Most days, I can recognize the reality of Molly's being ill, getting worse, never getting any better. Still, Molly is not in immanent danger of dying.

I personally, however, am much better. I have survived cancer treatment and am cancer-free now. I have completed my Fourth and Fifth Steps in my Twelve Step program and am well along on my Sixth. I have studied Buddhism. I have completed the year-long Course in Miracles. I have started therapy again. I am healthier physically, emotionally, socially, psychologically, and spiritually.

As Molly's illness has progressed, her health has gotten much worse. Her memory is truly gone. There are no flashes of childhood as is often the case with other Alzheimer's patients.

Something, obvious to everyone but me, is the fact that I was so busy taking care of Molly and others in my family that I never spent time or energy or money on myself. I was always at the bottom of the list and sometimes not even *on* the list.

My tools for fashioning a healthier me are not too complicated: I meditate every day. I write about my experiences (including taboo subjects like sex, death, and incontinence). I share my emotions with trusted friends, especially in my Twelve Step program (I just celebrated twenty-four years there). I do my sharing at meetings and, even more often, on the phone. I go to therapy and use the opportunity to let go of past baggage and deal with current stress.

I listen to music that suits my moods, including upbeat songs when I am feeling low. I take naps. I take pictures. I visit my grandchildren and let my inner child come out to play with them.

With Molly and the facility, I have adapted to the "new normal" as things changed: Molly's everyday condition and crises, the departures and arrivals of staff members, the deaths of some of my favorite residents and the absence of their caregivers who had become my friends.

At long last, I have come to understand that there is no such thing as "normal" with Alzheimer's. There is only change, and decline. Every day is different: every visit is different.

Now my visits are less frequent. In the first year, I could tell you that in nine months I had missed visiting on exactly thirty-three days. I don't keep track like that anymore, and I don't feel guilty about days I miss.

I don't get triggered in the same way. I don't feel guilty when Molly falls asleep and I leave (I used to wait for her to wake up again). I don't feel guilty when I leave after Molly walks away from me to be with someone else. I don't feel abandoned when she just wanders off.

This is Molly now with Alzheimer's. This is not the Molly I have known for over thirty years nor the Molly I would like to see. Quite simply she is the way she is. I can deal with Molly just the way she is, or I can deny her illness or run away from it, but I cannot change it. Complete "acceptance" and peace is still elusive and may never come, yet I am coping much better now.

Ultimately I have learned one of the key lessons of life: I cannot change anyone else, but I can change myself. I am different now. I have new interests, new friends, new directions. I am very much aware of not being half of the couple we were for so long. To have a life as a person separate from Molly is sometimes sad, but my life is also very exciting.

I have come a long, long way from the suicidal, self-pitying sad sack who wept in desperate loneliness after leaving Molly at the facility.

I am glad to be alive.

SELF-CARE CONTINUED

In my Al-Anon Twelve Step group, the leader of the meeting is asked to speak from his or her own "experience, strength, and hope." What it boils down to is "I have been through tough situations. I have not only survived but I have also grown from the challenges I faced. I am no different from you. If I can do it, so can you."

This past summer, I tested this premise in a whole new way, a thoroughly physical way. I joined a hiking group that climbs mountains in Colorado. I have long been a mountain *hiker* but never, ever thought of myself as a mountain *climber*. I was then 64 years old with one repaired knee, and thought I would never climb a 14er (14,000 foot+ peak).

But the people I was with have been doing this for twenty-five years. They know how to build up your stamina and your breathing to climb the high mountains. So, I did nine hikes with them and ended the summer climbing two 13ers and two 14ers before my 65th birthday.

And I started to get "I can't" out of my vocabulary.

With Molly and her Alzheimer's, I had many, many I can't moments. I can't find her: she's wandered off, and I don't know where she is. I can't reach her: she's having a psychotic episode. I can't get her to take a shower today: she is afraid of the water.

Finally, there was the moment of decision: I can't take care of Molly at home anymore and keep her healthy and safe. She needs to go into a facility where there are trained staff who can care for her 24-7.

After Molly went into the memory-care facility, I hit a big I can't. "I can't go on. I have no purpose in life now that my job as a full-time caregiver has ended. I don't know how to do anything else other that care for my loved ones."

"I certainly can't take care of myself. I don't know how. I just can't go on. I might as well just take a bottle of pills and go to sleep."

Obviously, that scenario did not play out. I am still here. I have, in the last year and a half, learned *how to take care of myself.*

Finally: Did I have to wait until I reached bottom to learn how to take care of myself? Perhaps. Regardless, I know now that effective self-care is *possible* whatever the circumstances. I could have done *some* of these things while Molly was still at home.

Self-care is doable. I am worth it. You are worth it.

DENIAL OF DEATH

March 24, 2014

I have bronchitis and sinusitis from a bad cold, so I haven't been able to visit Molly. I asked one of the nurses to tell me how she is doing: "She's been doing well. Molly seems quite happy: today she was walking around the building and playing with the hems of her dresses. She still dozes off throughout the day, but she lets us help her eat, and she sits in activities and watches or sits in the living room with other residents."

This description of "doing well" set me off, for sure. That's it? She's still able to walk? She's getting pleasure from wearing a dress again? She sits and watches activities she can't do anymore? That counts as doing well?

From the nurse's point of view that may be so, but it is not very good from my perspective. I want something more. I want some part of the old Molly to be there—to manifest. Rather I want to hear: She smiles. She laughs at jokes. She sings along when music plays. She displays some enthusiasm for her favorite foods: she likes it when they have chocolate chip cookies.

I don't want her to be merely walking, dozing, sitting, and being fed, yet often that's all there is to her day.

I sure don't get what *I* want. Alzheimer's wins every time. The disease is in charge, not me. I just get to be frustrated, angry, confused, and sad—still very sad sometimes.

Until I can be with her and hold her hand and sing to her and, I hope, sing with her. Then I'll feel better again. Until the next round of seizures and the inevitable decline that follows.

I still go up and down emotionally after years of this.

In my Twelve Step program, we are encouraged to "detach with love." In the Buddhist tradition I follow, we strive to let go of all attachments. We learn that nothing is permanent. Everything changes, and human beings, in particular, get old and sick and then they die.

I hear the lessons to be learned. I know—as they say "in my head"—that this is true. No matter what happened to Molly, she was, in the course of time, going to age and weaken and eventually die. She is turning 76. When I was first aware of life expectancies, that age was considered near the average endpoint for women, regardless of health or circumstances.

So what is going on in my brain and in my heart? Why resist what is? Why worry and suffer when nothing—and I mean nothing—can be done?

It is certainly human to fear death and to pretend that it happens to others but not to yourself and to those you love. Maybe it's as simple as that: we know the truth, but we have learned to deny what is unpleasant or uncomfortable or painful. Supposedly, that is the only way that women ever have a second child after the pain of labor.

Finally, the last stage of the grieving process is supposed to be acceptance not denial. Perhaps I only think I have grieved the loss of Molly, the Molly I knew and loved for thirty years. In January 2014, Molly was supposedly close to death and was put on hospice. It was a false alarm, yet it was deeply traumatic. I was an emotional wreck.

Now I'm afraid I have more ups and downs to come.

Today I'm not at all peaceful in the face of Molly's death. I'm scared and sad and angry.

Calm acceptance will have to wait.

DOES SHE KNOW YOU?

There are two perpetually recurring questions from relatives and friends?
"How is she?" "Does she know who you are?"

I believe both reflect the deepest fears we all share about our loved ones
when they are sick—"How sick is she? Is she dying?" And when they have
memory loss—"Will she still know me? Will there still be a bond between
us?"

Using the Alzheimer's Association definition of the phases of the disease,
Molly is at stage six of seven. She walks unsteadily and is at greater risk of
falling. She struggles to do simple things like getting up from a chair: she has
to find the arms of the chair and figure out how to push herself up. This
movement is no longer automatic for her.

Her attention span is much, much shorter than it was before the seizures six
months ago. She can get distracted between spoonfuls of food while I am
feeding her lunch. When we walk around inside the building—where she has
lived for almost two years—she can lose track of which way to turn to get to
her room. When I take her in the car, she forgets how to get out when we
arrive at the ice cream parlor.

I think of her now as disabled in a way I never did before. She needs help
with virtually every activity of daily living. It is terribly sad and sometimes
frightening to see how far she has declined. Yet, her fundamental health is
good. Barring a catastrophic fall that breaks her hip or a serious bout of
pneumonia, she may live for years.

Question two: "Does she recognize you?"

"What do you mean? Of course she does. She *has* to know the sound of
my voice. She's heard it for thirty years. She *has* to know my face. We
human beings are very, very good at face recognition. It's part of what
makes us human. We know our mother's face, our little sister's face, our
best friend's face. It's what we do every time we enter a room. 'Do I know
anyone here? Oh good, there's cousin Patty.'"

"When she makes eye contact, she has to know the look in my eyes. She has to know the touch of my hand in hers. She has to know the feel of my fingers brushing the hair from her forehead. She has to *know me.*"

"Of course, she recognizes me."

"Or does she?"

Actually, I don't really know. Do I? How can I possibly know what's still there? How can I know what the remaining neurotransmitters in her brain can still process, and what has been forgotten forever. There's no way to really know, no way to be sure.

I can only wish or hope or long for the instant of knowing. Yes, she does still know who I am. Yes, I am still important to her. Yes, I still mean something to her. Yes, I still exist for her.

We are still close. She knows I care for her and love her. She still loves me.

She is. I am. We are.

SENSE OF HUMOR

One of the primary things we human beings use to describe one another is sense of humor. We're hardwired to recognize strangers as friends or foes. Within our tribe we identify people with "She's great fun to be with: she has a wonderful sense of humor." Or, "My boss is impossible: he just has no sense of humor!"

Molly has always had a quite well-developed sense of humor. She saw the laughable absurdities in life all the time. She loved humorous literature of all kinds, from Edward Lear's nonsense poems to Shakespeare's puns.

We reserved a special reverence for Oscar Wilde, our pick as the funniest writer ever in the English language. We often quoted from his play, *The Importance of Being Earnest,* and we laughed every time:

"I was married once. It was the result of a misunderstanding between myself and a young person."
"It creates a false impression. That is just what dentists do."
"French songs are so vulgar . . . German sounds a respectable language, and I believe is so."
"Do you smoke?" "Yes, Lady Bracknell, I do." "Good, a gentleman should always have an occupation."

This is just one example of Molly's brand of humor, which we shared over the years. Sharing humor was part of our daily routine of reading in bed before going to sleep at night. We'd almost always be reading different books, but when we got to a funny part, we'd invariably read it out loud to each other and laugh out loud together.

When we adopted D.J., he became part of the evening ritual of reading before bedtime. We read to him, and Molly and he created their own comic routine at the beginning of "Peter Rabbit."

Molly (reading): "There were four little rabbits, Flopsie, Mopsie, Cottontail, and P. . .
D.J. (interrupting): "Benjamin."
Molly (emphatically) "No Benjamin Bunny!"

They'd repeat this several times until they both broke down into giggling laughter.

Molly had a wonderful, active, comprehensive sense of humor. Everyone who knew her would have agreed to that. What about now? Is there anything left of that part of her brain where humor resides?

I'd say, "Yes." For one thing, she still laughs. She laughs when I make silly faces at her, and, today, she was making silly faces back at me. She laughs at the antics of some of her fellow residents. Today she laughed a lot.

I like to cling to whatever I see is still left of the Molly I've known for decades. "Oh, yes, I recognize her laughter. She is still here. She is still with me."

It's pretty clear that that is my perception and my desire, perhaps my fantasy. Molly's reality is different, and who knows if she laughs now at the same kind of jokes and absurdities that tickled her before.

However, the good news is that, in the moment when I bug out my eyes and she laughs, what remains of her sense of humor isn't important. We share the moment. It is fun for both of us. I can be very happy with that much.

TOUCH IS LOVE PART 2

Molly had a lucid period last week, and I missed it, which seems very unfair. One of the newer caregivers "had a conversation" with her for the first time. I haven't had a conversation with Molly beyond "Do you want to go outside?" "Uh-huh." in over a year.

I'd love to know what she said, what she is aware of, how she thinks and feels at this point. Ironically I missed the opportunity. Maybe it will happen again when I am present.

Molly did communicate with me using words a couple of days ago. We were walking around the outside of the building, and she had stopped to look at a tree. When she turned to go on, Molly bumped into me. She said, "Oops, sorry."

I was thrilled. She spoke. She made sense. She can still talk. This is great.

That was the extent of her conversation for that day, but it was remarkably uplifting.

I think I can honestly say that I have no expectations when I go to see her now. She may be asleep and unresponsive. She may be unable or unwilling to walk around. She may not want to eat whatever I am trying to feed her. She probably won't join in when I sing to her.

So, how do she and I handle visits? I try, as much as possible, to sense her energy and moods and just be with her wherever she is that day. She seems to want to connect. She makes eye contact; she smiles; she touches me.

We hold hands much of the time we are together. Molly will sometimes initiate by reaching for my hand. She has also, on more than one occasion, explored my fingers and thumb as though feeling them for the first time. She will also stroke my hand and arm and other parts of my body. It is quite clear that this is connecting for her, and I take it as a great compliment.

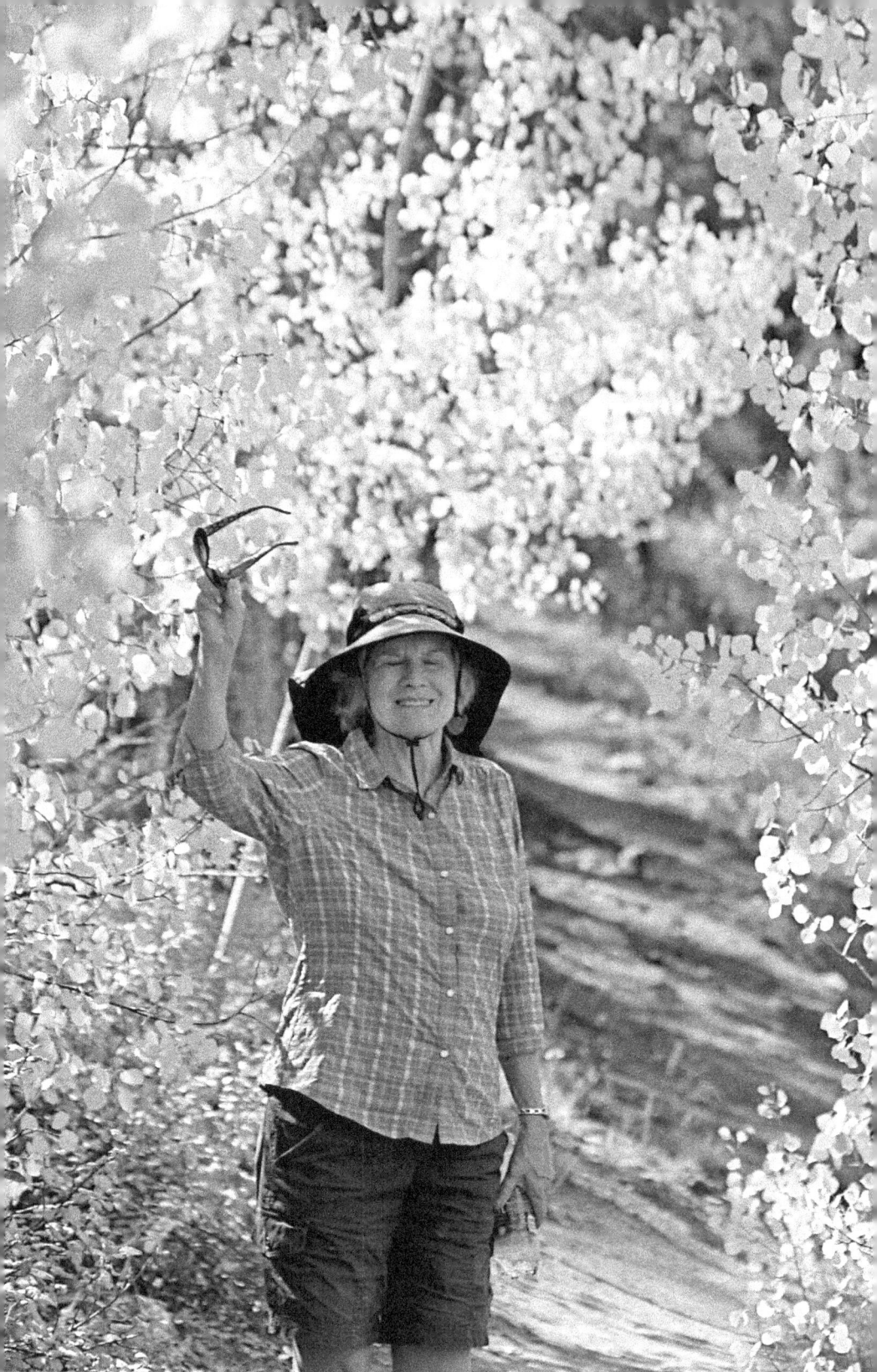

Molly at Twin Lakes, Colorado, amongst the fall aspens.

The look in her eyes, her smile, and her touch all say "I love you" when there are no words left. Today, that is more than enough for me.

TWO YEARS!

September 10, 2014

Today marks two years since I took Molly to the facility.

The anniversary brings back powerful memories of the "beginning." How I wept in grief.

How Molly reacted with anger and agitation. How she looked in every room in the place to see if she could find me. How the Director was freaked out by Molly's aggressive behavior.

How deep I was in guilt and shame and despair. How angry I was with an unjust God. How my friends Beth and Karl took me in and kept me safe for a week of terrible days and nights. How I considered suicide. How I awoke to life.

How the staff kept me from seeing Molly for seventeen days even though the policy was three weeks. How I snuck into the conference room and watched the back of Molly's head through a window. How I woke up alone in our bed every morning and always slept on "my side." How I learned to cook meals for one instead of two. How I filled my days and nights with activities and people so I wouldn't have to face being alone with myself.

How my friends and family rallied around me. How I made new friends. How I started to learn new things. How Molly's life changed forever. How my life changed forever.

This writing actually started months after Molly's placement, when I first traveled by myself to visit my sister Bernadette in California. Bern was teaching an adult education class on caregiving for the elderly (there are no accidents in life) at Leeza's Place in Los Angeles. The three Leeza's Place centers (in Florida, Illinois, and California) where founded by the TV personality Leeza Gibbons. Her mother had died of Alzheimer's, and she recognized the great need for programs to help those doing the difficult and exhausting work of caring for a loved one with memory loss.

So, about ten weeks after my "I can't do this anymore" crisis, I found myself telling my story to Stefanie, the Director of Leeza's Place. She listened attentively and asked questions for about an hour. Then she said, "You know, we have a lot of trouble getting men involved in our programs. We have almost all women come here. . . . I don't want to give you anything else to do, but if you ever had anything to share about your experiences it could be helpful to other men."

That night—fired by three cups of coffee—I wrote my first essay "I am a man and I am a caregiver."

My sister Jamie, a singer, producer, and artists' coach, showed that first essay to Zoe, a well-published writer friend who had retired from teaching at Columbia College in Chicago. Zoe's response to that piece was, in part, "You're writing a book." "I can't do that," I said, "I might be able to write ten newspaper columns on Tips for Caregivers, but I could never write a book." "I think you have about three books in you. But we'll start with this one." Zoe also told me that her first principle for teaching/coaching writers was no judgments on first drafts. "Just keep writing and sending the work to me."

So I did. I most often wrote at night recounting the events of the day or week. I'd sleep on it, edit the text the next morning, and send it to Zoe as an e-mail attachment.

Over time I have been much concerned, even obsessed, with memory and memories: Molly's losing hers and my preserving mine and hers. Over the years Molly shared stories about her family and her life that no one else remembers now. I am the only one, and it is both an honor and a source of pain to hold Molly's life in my mind and heart.

As I was writing this, I became aware that this writing—these stories and essays—have captured our memories over the last two years.

For one thing, Molly has a new extended family, all the residents she lives with and the caregivers who help her with Activities of Daily Living. At one point I decided to think of them all as her new "cousins."

Molly's also had some "special friends," men she hung out with and had some attachment to. All of those male friends are gone now, either moved to skilled nursing or dead.

Some of my favorite residents have died as well. Still I remember all of them, and I have the written record of some of the moments Molly and I shared with them. These are precious memories, and I am very glad to have saved them.

MARRIAGE VOWS

September 14, 2014

After thirty years, I honestly can't remember exactly what vows Molly and I used at our wedding, but I'm sure they were some version of the traditional:

"I, Willem, take you Molly, to be my wife, to have and to hold from this day forward, for better or for worse, for richer, for poorer, in sickness and in health, to love and to cherish; from this day forward until death do us part."

I was reminded of the vows yesterday at the wedding of my niece. I was there without Molly, of course. There is no way she could travel anymore.

"In sickness and in health" resonates these days in a deep and powerful way. In fact, it comes up every time I visit, every time I get a call that something has happened to her, every time someone asks, "How is Molly doing?" I've written before about my response to the Billy Joel song "I Love You Just the Way You Are." It makes me cry every time: I love Molly in her sickness, and I grieve the loss of Molly's health.

I have actually recited the wedding vows twice. The first time was with Sharon, from whom I was divorced after twelve years. The "until death" part didn't happen, and it was pretty unlikely since I was a very naïve 22 at the time. I had no clue about a relationship, much less a forever marriage. So I can cut myself a break on that one, especially since Molly and I have now passed our thirtieth anniversary.

With Molly, however, there's also "until death do us part." At the basic level that vow is still unshakeable. I have heard of people getting divorces at the end of life for financial reasons, but I don't see that happening with me and Molly. I fully expect that we will indeed be married until death do us part.

That would be what most people would call the "letter" of the vow. The presumed "spirit" of the vow is that I would not have another romantic partner while Molly is alive.

Some of my closest friends and family have weighed in on this issue, "Molly would never have wanted you to be lonely and to not have love in your life. And, if the positions were reversed, wouldn't you want Molly to be happy with someone?" Sure I would.

And I am not alone. I read an article recently about married caregivers who get involved with other caregivers, even one case where the newly formed couple share care for their spouses with dementia. It seems that many caregivers in my position find romance and comfort and affection and, yes, sex outside of marriage.

The person I married is not there anymore. We live apart. She makes attachments with other residents. As rationalization goes, this is pretty good: both the Molly would want you to be happy part, and the old Molly is gone part.

Have I actively sought a new relationship? Yes. Do I still feel guilty sometimes? Sure.

Am I happy with my partner? Very happy. Would Molly wish me happy? Yes.

Part Four: Meditations

DEATH AND REBIRTH

What is continually surprising to me is that the story of Molly, me, and Alzheimer's is just as much about my dying as Molly's. Hers is a physical death due to a devastating illness. Mine is an emotional, psychological, and spiritual death and subsequent rebirth and new life.

Losing the Molly I knew and loved was beyond anything I had experienced. For years, I hid from grief by staying very busy taking care of her 24/7. I followed her around the house and kept sharp objects on a high shelf; I installed a special locking device on the top of the front door so she couldn't get out and wander away; I eventually did all of the driving—sometimes just going where she pointed; I bought a new washer and dryer with a sanitary cycle to clean her clothing when she began to be incontinent; I read to her when she could no longer read herself; I cooked all the meals when she could no longer remember to turn off the stove; and so on.

It worked up to a point. I put affirmations from tips for Alzheimer's patients up on the refrigerator: "Learn new things." "Eat fish." "Exercise." "Don't accept decline as inevitable." Molly said to Nancy, a close friend, "It doesn't hurt, you know." I thought, "This is better than a painful death from cancer or losing a limb to diabetes."

Actually I was the one who got the cancer. I was diagnosed with prostate cancer in 2010 and had successful surgery in 2011. (Today I am cancer free with a non-detectible PSA.) Was the cancer brought on by the stress of Molly's illness and caring for her? Perhaps, but I do know that cancer runs in my family so it may well be just a coincidence.

It was during my recovery from surgery that I first asked for help taking care of Molly. Even I, the dedicated, even fanatically attentive husband could not do everything all the time any more.   So I asked for help, and I got it. I consider learning to ask for help the true lesson of my cancer. First we got help from friends and family and later through a home care agency. Molly is very fortunate to have purchased long-term care insurance before she retired, and in-home respite care was covered under her policy.

I took Molly to the facility on September 10, 2012. I was not allowed to see Molly for three weeks while she adjusted to her new surroundings and new caregivers.

I stayed with Beth and her husband Karl for a week and returned home on my birthday September 17th. For the next two days, I was in the grip of a deep depression that led to "suicidal ideation," as the psychiatric community labels it.

I was done with life, without a purpose, alone and miserable. I was also completely exhausted from the full-out effort of the previous five years. Bern said to me, "Willem, you have 2% left: you are going to have to do something about Molly's care."

Thus I (perhaps melodramatically) believe I died on September 19, 2012.

Of course, I didn't really die. On the morning of the 20th, I awoke with the realization, "I am still here. What the hell am I going to do now?"

Change my life and become a different person in many ways: Change my thinking and behavior, learn new things, develop new friendships, work on my Twelve Steps, take A Course in Miracles, begin to practice Buddhist meditation. All of the above.

And very significantly write this book, which describes my thoughts and feelings as I have been going through the process of Molly's path towards death and my journey of rebirth and reinvention.

Molly's body is still alive, although her cognitive and physical abilities are much compromised. I, however, have not only been able to cope with my beloved's terminal illness but also to grow from the experience.

WHAT NOW?

My sister Jamie, in her role as artists' coach, asked me about the title of this book, "Maybe it should be a question."

The question that immediately popped into my mind was "Why?" But upon sleeping and dreaming on it, a better question arose: "What do I do now?"

I have asked that question over and over during the Alzheimer's years. Often, I asked it of Bernadette and Stefanie, who were my go-to experts. "Molly just did this." or "This just happened for the first time." "What do I do now?"

That was the daily life version, but there was another "What now?" This question arose the morning I awoke after considering ending my life. I realized I was still alive, and I had no idea what came next. "I am still here. What the hell do I do now?!"

I was fortunate to have been among friends who actually had good suggestions. "Why don't you come with me to the Buddhist group meditation and dharma talk tonight." "You could finish your Al-Anon Fourth Step and do a Fifth Step." "How about joining the Course in Miracles class: it would be good for you to be around people who believe in a God of Love."

Karl also told me about his encounters with people who had had near-death experiences. He described, in detail, one woman's story about meeting God and being shown a mass of human faces. She got the message that if she decided to return to life, she would help the vast number of people spread out before her. The woman decided to return, and, when she met Karl, she recognized him as one of the faces she had seen in her vision.

When I was a student, I thought existentialist philosophy was really cool. We are responsible for our lives because we are constantly making choices that matter. We get to make the biggest choice of all: to live or die.

I faced my own such choice when I took Molly to the facility. Was my life over once I lost my caretaking purpose for living? If not, then what lessons did I have yet to learn, how would I change and grow moving forward? What was I to do with the next twenty years or more?

Two years later, I have some experience of life beyond caretaking. I have had the extraordinary opportunity to reinvent myself at age 64, to start fresh and choose a much more wholehearted life, a life that includes not just what I have to do or what others expect me to do. I get to really and truly ask, "What do I want to do? What am I passionate about? What do I want to learn?"

Yes, I have been grieving Molly's losses and my losses. But beyond the grieving—I would say *way* beyond the grieving—I have been opening up to a new life I could not have imagined.

Ultimately, today my life journey yields a new answer to the question "What do I do now?" "I live more fully and completely, and I write about my life. I write about both what has been lost and what I have discovered."

FIELD OBSERVER

My friend Lee recently asked me about how the symptoms of Alzheimer's compare with those of other types of dementia. I had trouble answering. I've done some studying of dementia in general and Alzheimer's in particular, but I am in no way an expert.

When in comes to Alzheimer's, I now subscribe to the notion that "When you know an Alzheimer's patient, you know *one* Alzheimer's patient." There just is no general description that fits all, or even the majority of, cases.

Though I am not an expert, I am an experienced Alzheimer's observer. After all, I had visited Molly some 300 times in the first year. My direct observations keep reminding me that human beings behave in surprising ways. This is true with and without the disease.

I have, for example, witnessed behavior in Alzheimer's patients that reflects the will to live and the will to die. There is one woman who lived at the facility for a couple of years and, eventually, was taken home by her husband when she was near death. Despite the reasonable predictions of her doctor and hospice nurse, she is still alive. More than a year after everyone, except her, expected her to die, there she was with her husband at the staff appreciation dinner this summer.

In another case one of the male patients had a reputation for bothering the females with his amorous attentions. Reggie was still full of the life force. I mostly admired his energy and didn't begrudge the time that Molly spent hanging out with him. Last month, I noticed that Reggie was not at lunch, and I asked one of the care partners about him. I was told that he had stopped eating, that he was lying in bed in his room, and that he was expected to pass away soon. Reggie is gone now. How or why he decided not to eat and to let go of his powerful life force remains a mystery.

One thing that is interesting to me about these two cases is how differently two patients with similar diagnostic profiles acted. In the old days, people talked about will power as applying to many aspects of life, like quitting smoking or losing weight or giving up alcohol. Nowadays, it appears that such life choices are more complicated. It's not just will power but an inexplicable combination of DNA and family background and socio-economics and many other factors that determine human behavior. This complex mix of factors makes it hard or impossible to predict what anyone will do.

Shakespeare memorably summarized the ultimate test of human will as "To be or not to be?" Is someone with an Alzheimer's-damaged brain still able to ask and answer that question? It would seem so.

If that is true, then what else is going on in the Alzheimer's patient's mind? Alzheimer's is at once a heartbreaking and a fascinating disease.

GRIEF AND THE SPIRITUAL PATH

According to different spiritual traditions, there are various ways of defining ultimate human peace and joy, such as enlightenment/awakening, heaven, divine union, the Kingdom, or Christ consciousness.

In no way can I claim to be enlightened. However I have progressed spiritually in the last few years. And I believe my spiritual path is directly interconnected with the emotional journey of grieving.

In my case, of course, it is "anticipatory" grieving, since Molly—however absent she may be—is still alive.

The classic formulation of the grieving process was developed by Elisabeth Kübler-Ross, who identified five stages: denial, anger, bargaining, depression, and acceptance. I relate to her understanding though I am still waiting for acceptance. Maybe full acceptance is like enlightenment: it is a goal nobly to be sought without any expectation of reaching it.

In the Buddhist tradition, enlightenment is possible although it may well take many lifetimes. According to the fundamental teaching of the Four Noble Truths, all human beings need to face the reality that: 1. Life is suffering. 2. Grasping, clinging, craving, and desire all cause suffering. 3. Cessation of suffering is possible. 4. The Eightfold Path is the spiritual path leading to the cessation of suffering or awakening or enlightenment. The Buddha taught that, by *abandoning desire in all its forms,* the skillful means to a cessation of suffering can be developed.

No desire for anything, including love, happiness, health, or success for one's children, is a pretty tall order. Thus there is a new hypothesis in contemporary Buddhist teachings. If we cannot reach absolute enlightenment, absent all human needs and wants, is there some consolation? Maybe. There is Noble Truth 3.5: suffering can be managed.

Under this rubric, when we experience a painful loss, we can grieve and recover without complete acceptance/enlightenment. As long as we face and accept our feelings, however unpleasant, and don't try to avoid or suppress them, we can live full and happy lives.

I'm currently in this camp. It is still very painful to see Molly in decline and more and more disabled by her illness. I don't think I will ever truly feel that it is fair that this brilliant, good woman should suffer from this terrible disease.

Yet I don't have to be stuck in denial or anger or bargaining or depression. I can choose to live with a measure of peace and be open to the joys of life, even without Molly by my side.

It's not at all what I wanted, and sometimes I hate the fact that she is no longer there. However, I am alive and well, and that is something to be grateful for every day.

LETTING GO AND HOLDING ON

I considered using "letting go" in the title since so much of this time has been about letting go of Molly, letting go of being half of a couple, letting go of my caregiver life, and, later on, letting go of my old self in emotional and spiritual ways.

"Let go and let God" is one of the key slogans of my weekly Twelve Step meetings. In my Buddhist meditation classes and practice, we focus on letting go of all attachments as essential to the path towards peace and enlightenment.

I understand the wisdom of these principles, and I have benefited from following them. Yet there is a part of me that wants to hold on. I especially want to hold onto the memories of my life with Molly over the last thirty years. I want to hold onto the photographs that document those memories, the souvenirs of our trips together, the letters and cards from friends and family, the birthday and Christmas gifts, the drawings by our children inscribed with "I love you, Mom." "I love you, Dad."

I recently moved and faced downsizing our, now my, stuff in a major way. In some cases, I found a lovely way to hold onto the memories and let go of the stuff. I gave it away, both to family members who will appreciate the connection and to thrift stores where people will make good use of it. "Here is a piece of jewelry we bought on a trip to the Southwest over twenty years ago. Use it and have fun." "Here is a cookbook Molly used. I hope you will enjoy the recipes your Grandma Molly made." "This book of poems was one of your Aunt Molly's favorites. Read them and enjoy." The young recipients have all responded with surprise and delight. I am sure Molly would be pleased.

Of course the memories stored in my heart are much more important than any object or photo. I have an almost infinite number of these treasures. I know they will always be with me.

Yet I still fear losing the memories as I age. Molly has no memories left. I may well reach that stage myself at some point. It seems scary and lonely to be without the traces of past experiences that were beautiful and precious. I meditate to appreciate the present moment. I do believe that the present moment is the only time that is real. The past is indeed gone away. The future is completely unknown and unknowable.

When I am actually with Molly rather than thinking of her, I can sometimes get into the present with her. She seems to be in the present all of the time. I can join her in the moment when I am aware. Then I am truly holding her hand and feeling the touch of her skin on mine. I am truly looking into her eyes as she first makes eye contact when I visit. I truly feel the warmth of her smile.

It is not the smile of the past. It is not captured in a photograph.

In that moment, I let go without struggle. My thoughts disappear, and I simply smile.

LESS IS MORE

September 30, 2014

Often when I'm half awake in the morning, messages from my unconscious mind come through. This morning the message was "You can get better by not trying so hard to get better."

As a life-long perfectionist, I always try really, really hard. This morning, I realized that I have been taking self-care to a whole new level. It's not hard to understand. Over the last few years, I've gotten two questions from friends and family and professionals and well-meaning strangers: "How is Molly doing?" and "What are you doing to take care of yourself?"

I've got a long list with which to answer the second question I meditate; I hike to stay fit; I cook meals from scratch; I go to Twelve Step meetings; I go to two book clubs; I study A Course in Miracles; I spend time with friends; I go to therapy. . . I often have three or four or, even, five things scheduled in a single day. I have six self-help books on my night table, and yesterday I bought two more!

Enough.

In one of those self-help books, *The Gifts of Imperfection*, author Brene Brown says, "We convince ourselves that if we stay busy and keep moving, reality won't be able to keep up. So we stay in front of the truth about how tired and scared and confused and overwhelmed we sometimes feel."

I also live in Boulder, Colorado, AKA the People's Republic of Boulder, where there are unlimited opportunities to stay busy with classes, lectures, workshops, healings, performances, art exhibits, films, and events. I have many things in a given week that are stimulating or entertaining or social or inspiring or growth promoting. After putting my life on hold for years to care for Molly, I am the kid in a candy store. I want it all, right now, and tiredness be damned. Take a nap. Drink coffee. Go on to the next thing.

None of this is surprising. Molly's illness and decline is often scary and confusing and overwhelming. Of course, I distract myself when I can.

But I've also had the experience of burnout in caring for Molly, and I don't want to repeat it in caring for myself.

So, today, I have a new awareness of what I have been doing for the past two years. It's been enjoyable, and I have grown tremendously. But I don't have to be a perfectionist about myself. I can choose a different path this time.

My life task is not to be a better and better person until I finally get to be the perfect person I imagine I want to be or whom others expect me to be. My task is to let go of trying so hard and to accept who and what I am. I'm the only one who thinks I am flawed or imperfect. The Universe sees me as whole, complete, and beautiful just as I am.

This is going to be challenging and require some significant changes in the ways I feel, think, and act; but it can be done.

I can learn to take even better care of myself.

Let go. Say no. Relax. Be still.

That sounds pretty darn good.

STOP AND WATCH THE SUNSET

This evening, I was on my way to chorus practice. It was towards the end of rush hour, and there was still heavy traffic and lots of red lights. I was particularly annoyed with a car ahead of me traveling five miles slower than the speed limit. To get to the rehearsal space, I go due west towards the foothills of the Rockies. The sun was just setting, and the clouds were mostly gray when I started out. Soon, however, a spectacular sunset began to paint the clouds a brilliant orange. This display lasted many minutes before the coloring changed to a bright pink against the color that defines sky blue.

All of a sudden, I laughed out loud. "Here God is giving you extra time to enjoy this incredible light show, and all you want to do is complain about the traffic."

Molly would never get so distracted from the present moment.

Today we walked around outside the building where she lives. Molly was energetic and created her own route. At one point, she left the sidewalk and headed into the adjoining landscaping. To my surprise, Molly said, "Let's go this way." Then she simply marched right over some short shrubs that were between her and where she was headed.

Molly encountered some rose bushes and felt one of the thorns prick her finger. She reacted with a strong "Ooh" as she withdrew her hand from the offending bush. A few minutes later, Molly came up to another rosebush and shook her hand as though reacting again to a thorn pricking her. Whatever the capacity of her short-term memory, she remembered what she needed to know about roses and thorns.

Over the weekend I was talking with my friend Jackie about Molly's regressing and often behaving like a small child just learning about the world. My friend Jackie wisely answered, "Just think of all the things she has to teach you."

Some lessons from today then:

Make your own path through life. There is no need to stick to the sidewalk that someone else laid down.

Don't be afraid to take on challenges. You are stronger and more capable than you think.

A little pain is no big deal if you learn from the experience.

Pay attention to what is before you right now instead of worrying about where you're going next.

Otherwise you might miss the best sunset of the year.

MOLLY'S TRUE SELF

Life Lessons by Elizabeth Kübler-Ross and David Kessler contains a wonderful chapter on the ultimate question, "Who am I?" They say we can begin to identify our authentic selves if we observe people at the beginning and the end of life.

Most of us spend most of our lives playing roles given to us by our parents, our teachers, our bosses, our partners, our society. We become very good at playing the polite and obedient child, the cooperative student, the hard-working employee, the considerate spouse, and the good neighbor. Still we have little or no sense of who we really are under these facades. We're so busy doing what others expect us to do that we don't have time or space to explore what we truly want and need.

The authors believe that young children haven't yet learned the rules set by others nor what gets rewarded or punished in the family and the world. Consequently, they act out of what they truly feel and want. Similarly, those who are dying can finally drop the roles they have played all their lives. The young and the dying are most likely to think, feel, and behave authentically. They are our best role models and our best teachers.

I see the wisdom and the fundamental truth in this analysis. Yet, it is a challenge to my sense of Molly and our relationship.

Who was Molly before the onset of Alzheimer's? I thought she was first and foremost a brilliant scholar, a skilled writer, a dedicated teacher, a generous colleague, a loving wife, a dutiful daughter, a caring mother and grandmother, an active citizen, a stimulating companion, a perfect partner. Yes, she was all of these: she played all of the roles assigned to her really, really well.

I admired her for all of this and loved her for her many admirable qualities.

However, Kübler-Ross and Kessler suggest that what I thought I loved and admired was not the real, unchanging, true self of Molly. Rather, in many ways, the woman who nods off while I am with her, who sometimes walks away, who holds the hand of another, who says straight out "Don't do that" may well be more authentic than the person I thought I knew for thirty years.

Observing Molly now, I see a much more restless spirit, someone still willing to take risks, someone who lacks Overeaters Anonymous discipline when it comes to sweets, someone who finds comfort and companionship from more than one source, someone who labels all grandchildren as generic "little guys," someone who finds the texture of the curtains in her room much more fascinating than my conversation.

Which parts are the authentic Molly and which the Molly with the disease of Alzheimer's? Clearly, I don't know.

Yet I get it. I saw what I was trained to see and what I wanted to see and what Molly wanted the world to see. Molly was in every possible way a "good person." Does that mean that Molly had to be perfect, not a flawed human being living through the mistakes, changes, and surprises of life?

Maybe, underneath her public persona, Molly was sometimes selfish, proud, self-indulgent, addictive, and stubborn. That might make her less of a good person than I wanted her to be in *my* ideal world, but it surely didn't make her any less human, only more so.

And nothing made her less lovable.

Molly undoubtedly had a shadow side, like all humans do. Yet, her True Self was and is and always will be whole, perfect, and beautiful. That is infinitely beyond being "good.

NOT MOLLY'S HIGHER POWER

In the Twelve Step programs, we use the term Higher Power to refer to the spiritual essence that controls our lives. Most often we don't know or understand what is in our Higher Power's plan for us. Each of us, including Molly, has her or his own Higher Power. Molly's Higher Power cares for both her soul self and for her diseased body and brain.

That means that, at the deepest level, Molly doesn't need me to direct her life. Someone else is in charge, not I.

These thoughts came up for me today as I was feeding her lunch. The cooks, nutritionist, and nurses at Molly's facility have carefully planned the meals to provide all essential nutrients that the residents need. Today, Molly's lunch included chicken for protein, potatoes for fiber and carbohydrates, steamed squash for vitamins, and water and juice for fluids. In short, a complete and balanced meal.

Yet I, somehow thinking I am still responsible for Molly's health and well-being, was trying to control what she ate. I'd make sure I gave her some of the vegetables in between forkfuls of chicken or potatoes. I handed her the glass to make sure she drank enough water.

What was I thinking? That I still can act like I am Molly's sole caregiver and I am responsible for every aspect of her daily life?

Of course, I do want Molly to be as healthy and strong as she can be. All of the residents are ill, and many of them are quite old and frail. Yet their families and the staff are very concerned about their maintaining healthy habits. I was reminded of this preoccupation when I overheard this exchange:

Female Resident 1 (moving down the hall with her walker), "We sure do like to go around."
Female Resident 2, "Yes, it's our exercise."
Female Resident 1, "It's so healthy. It's good for us."

Evidently some ideas stick with us through thick and thin, even in dementia.

Back to me and Molly: Do I truly know what is good for her? Is there any sense in which I am really responsible for her well-being? Was I ever, or did I just think I was?

Today these seem like rhetorical questions. No one, not her doctors and certainly not I, had any way of knowing how Molly's individual case of Alzheimer's would develop: what medications she should have and for how long, what other medical issues she might have (her seizures, for example, are atypical for Alzheimer's), how long she would live.

Sometimes I would let the professionals take over and let the doctors, nurses, and care partners call the shots. Other times I'd resist them strongly, convinced that I needed to "advocate" for Molly on all parts of her care. Some of my advocacy may have been useful; some may have created unnecessary conflict between me and the pros.

Whatever the particulars, I am not Molly's Higher Power. Never was. Never will be.

I'm glad to have that insight, however long it took for the light to go on.

A STUDENT

October 31, 2014

I wrote at the outset about how this book started out to be about Molly and Alzheimer's. I wanted so desperately to understand what was going on and to have some answer—no matter how incomplete—to the question "Why?"

The writing changed as Molly declined and as I changed with grieving. I began to get positive feedback in several forms. The most common was admiration. "You are so dedicated to Molly's care. You are a wonderful and extraordinary person." Many people also commented on the value of my experiences and my willingness to write about them. "This will be so helpful to others."

I've already written about how I felt being called a "saint." How do I feel about being a role model for other caregivers? It's one more case of both/and: I know that my experiences have been typical in many ways of the anticipatory grief process. That makes me a good role model for others. On the other hand, my coping strategies are my own and not necessarily appropriate for others.

I have been an A student/perfectionist for most of my life. So it follows that I should strive to be a perfect caregiver and an A student at getting through my grief. I zealously studied A Course in Miracles, insight Buddhist meditation, and the Twelve Steps. I wanted to "get better" from grief and depression, and I thought I could do it with enough data and new skills.

What I was often really doing was running away, running away from sitting alone with my feelings. It was much too scary to watch Molly disappear and to start to live without her. It was really frightening to know, really know, that there is no cure for Alzheimer's and that Molly was going to die.

So I went to classes and meetings and events. I spent time with people in groups. I read and discussed and talked about everything new I was learning. I am a very good student and an articulate, educated person. I made friends and impressed them with my progress, my new attitude, my knowledge of emotional, psychological, and spiritual aspects of life.

I ran away fast and furious.

That's where I may not be a very good role model. For myself I needed to play out my grieving according to my perfectionist mindset. Clearly this is not for all caregivers. We dedicated caregivers can burn out even in our efforts to take care of ourselves. I know I've come pretty close to exhaustion doing what I and others thought was "good for me."

Thus I don't presume to recommend my path. It has worked for me so far. Will it work for anyone else? I cannot say.

FINAL THOUGHTS FOR CAREGIVERS

Whenever I mentioned that I was writing this book, I would get some version of this response, "Oh, this is so needed right now. Alzheimer's is everywhere. Your work will be so helpful to others who are dealing with the same things as you."

Here, in summary then, are some of my personal tools for becoming a healthier caregiver:

- Take naps to rest and re-charge.
- Listen to music that suits your moods, including upbeat songs when you are feeling low. I often sing along, especially in the car. When at home I often dance.
- Ask for help. You'll be pleasantly surprised to find that most everyone is willing to help out.
- Get regular exercise. My hiking is great in the summer. I use yoga classes and visits to the gym during the cold and snow of winter.
- Eat a healthy diet. I cook for myself even though I live alone. I find the cooking creative and therapeutic. It also offers immediate gratification. I get to eat the food, and it tastes good.
- Find a way to express your creativity. I take photos, and, of course, I write stories and poems.
- Spend time with children and let your inner child come out to play with them.
- Write about all your experiences, including taboo subjects like money, sex, death, and incontinence. No one else needs to see your grief journal.
- Share your emotions with trusted friends and family members. I especially find confidants in my Twelve Step program. I do my sharing at meetings and, even more often, on the phone.
- Meditate every day. Five to ten minutes a day makes a difference! I use a method called insight meditation. In this kind of meditation, one is not seeking a blank-minded blissful state but one is rather "mindful" of whatever comes up. For guidance in this practice, I recommend anything written by Thich Nhat Hanh.
- When the I-can't-meditate thoughts arise, just breathe deeply.
- Find a therapist and use the opportunity to let go of past baggage and cope more effectively with current stress.

Beyond a list of tips, I'd like offer this message to other Alzheimer's and dementia caregivers:

This is what happened to me: Molly, my wife of thirty years and my true soulmate, was diagnosed with Alzheimer's, a terrible disease that is terminal, untreatable, and incurable.

I was overwhelmed, angry with God and the Universe, alone in my grief, and suicidal. I got through it. I grew from the experience of caring for Molly as her mind disappeared. In the process I came to understand and appreciate my life as never before.

I am no different from you.

You can do it, too.

Choose to live fully and joyfully. Recognize how much strength and courage is already inside you. Know truly and deeply that you are never alone.

Always be grateful.

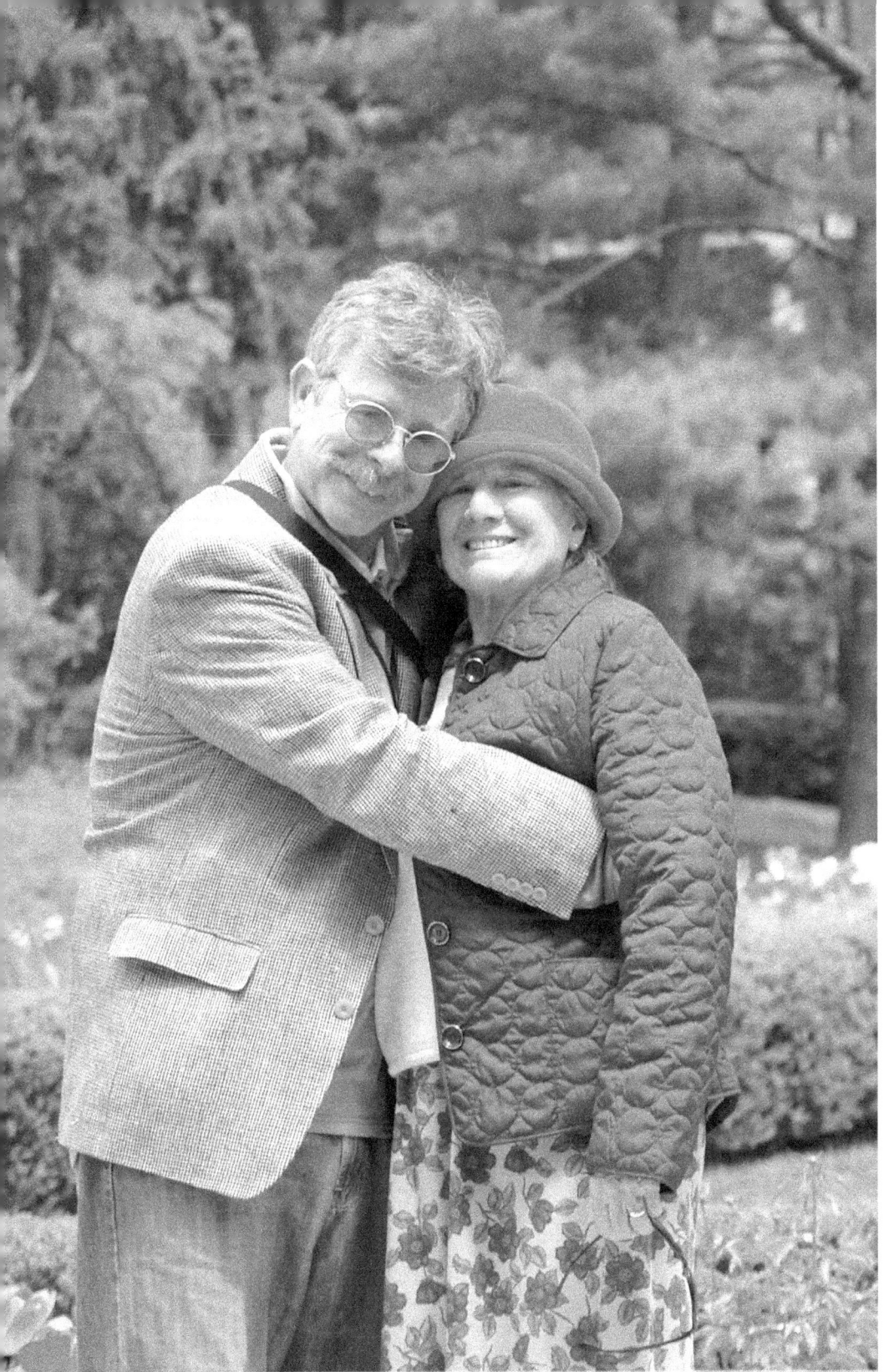

Molly and her husband Willem.

Notes

Notes

Notes

Notes

Willem O'Reilly is a freelance writer living in Colorado. Previously he was a college professor, a grant writer, a real estate agent, a tour guide, and a diversity trainer.

Over his career, Dr. O'Reilly has written everything from cartoon captions to multi-million dollar grant proposals. Dr. O'Reilly currently creates content for Internet businesses, including proposals, blogs, and online courses.

Together Willem and Molly have three grown children Mae 37, Reynor 36, and D.J. 35, who were adopted from the Philippines, and three grandchildren. Molly has three older children Cathy, Chris, and Nora and seven grandchildren.

Since writing this book, Willem has been sharing his experiences by speaking to support groups and others interested in Alzheimer's, caregiving, grief, and end-of-life.

Willem is available for discussions either in person or via Skype. Please contact him at willemor917writer.com

Acknowledgements

I am eternally grateful to

Molly's children and their spouses Cathy and Michael, Chris and Bethany, and Nora and Fred and our children and their spouses Mae and Rich, Reynor and Adrienne, and D.J.

Stefanie and Jackie and all of the angels and helpers, especially the kind and wonderful people who care for Molly every day.

My writing supporters: Alicia, Mary Ellen, Marilyn, Catherine, Jamie, Angelo, Adrienne, and Lee.

My Buddhist teachers: David, Johann, and Peter.

My A Course in Miracles brothers and sisters.

My Stephen Minister friend Jim.

My dear friends in recovery.

Willem is also a volunteer with the Speakers Bureau of the Alzheimer's Association of Colorado.

Willem is available to speak with your support, discussion, or book group in person or via Skype.

Please scan the code to visit my website for further information.
https://wordpress.com/willemor917writer.com

www.ingramcontent.com/pod-product-compliance
Lightning Source LLC
Chambersburg PA
CBHW021921020426
42334CB00013B/518